Original French edition:
"Le CANCER, un livre qui donne de l'espoir "
First printing: 2013
CAN ISBN 978-2-920932-56-2


First edition/First printing
National library of Canada
Bibliothèque et Archives nationales du Québec
ISBN 978-2-920932-70-8
Printed in Canada

**Worldwide print distributor**
Lotus Brands Inc.
P.O. Box 325
Twin Lakes, WI
53181 USA
Tel: 262-889-8501 or 1-800-824-6396
Fax: 262-889-2461
Email: lotuspress@lotuspress.com
www.lotuspress.com

**Publisher**
Les Editions E.T.C. Inc.
1102 Boul. La Salette
Saint-Jerome (Quebec)
J5L 2J7 Canada
Tel: 450-431-5336
Email: info@leseditionsetc.com
www.leseditionsetc.com

LISE BOURBEAU
BEST-SELLING AUTHOR OF
*"LISTEN TO YOUR BODY, your best friend on Earth"*

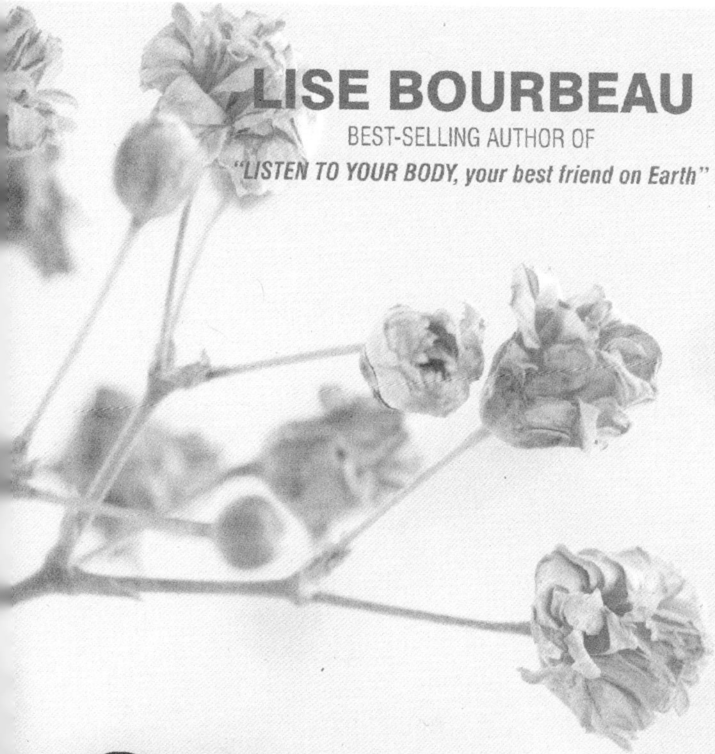

# Cancer
## A book of
## *Hope*

EDITIONS E.T.C. INC

# Table of contents

# Acknowledgments

THANK YOU to all *Listen to Your Body* workshop participants for being an inexhaustible source of real-life experiences, for continually reminding me about the amazing intelligence of this creation that is the human body, and for showing me that therefore anything is possible.

THANK YOU to those who have allowed me to cite their story in this book for the purpose of helping the general public.

THANK YOU especially to Denise, who agreed to let me use all the details of the forgiveness process she went through with her mother.

THANK YOU to everyone who encouraged me to write this book, especially my son-in-law, Jean-Pierre Gagnon – director of Éditions ETC – who first came up with the idea.

THANK YOU to my translator  Ferdinanda Van Gennip, who was most helpfull in the way she executed this task.

THANK YOU to all the doctors and therapists who are open to the idea that cancer can be cured by love, which encouraged me even more to write this book.

THANK YOU, dear readers, for being brave enough to undertake the experiences suggested in this book. I hope with all my heart that you will be able to contribute to improving the general statistics on cancer in the years to come.

# Prologue

It was in response to increasingly frequent questions about the causes of cancer and a suggestion made by my publisher that I decided to write a book on this subject. I know that several works, by very competent authors, have already been written on cancer. But what I want to share with you in this book is the synthesis that emerged from thirty years spent teaching the *Listen to Your Body* philosophy throughout the world.

Based on the testimonies of numerous people suffering from cancer who participated in the *LISTEN TO YOUR BODY School of Life* workshops, I gradually arrived at the conclusions appearing in this book.

I must admit that at first I hesitated for a long time, because the cause and origin of illnesses is such a broad and controversial topic. I know very well that ten years from now I will have learned still more. But I also know that I must not wait until I know everything before writing a book like this. In fact, it is impossible for us to know everything. That's the main reason I always want to keep on teaching. Teaching is undeniably my greatest source of new knowledge and discovery.

I have also learned much from several of my friends and family members who had cancer. Some of them were cured while others died from it. Frequently the examples you read in this book will be experiences gone through by many individuals. The names are fictitious, but the examples are real and of course all of the people in them have authorized me to share them with you.

I would like to point out that what you will be reading is the fruit of all my observations. I do not claim to possess the truth and my goal is not to convince anyone of everything that I have learned. I mainly wish to share those insights that made me go WOW, which were a tremendous help toward improving my own quality of life and that of so many others. My primary goal is to offer my testimony in the hope that whatever resonates with you will constitute a positive response to the needs of your soul.

You will note moreover that there is no bibliography at the end of this book and that very often I do not quote the source of what I have learned. I have actually been reading books on this subject for some forty years without necessarily jotting down all my sources. If you need proof, then you are reading with your 'mental body' and there is the risk that you are letting your ego take charge.

Any book on personal growth or spirituality should be read with the heart. This means taking the time to verify whether what you have just read leaves you with a good feeling. This attitude helps you develop discernment. You will be the person who makes the final decision as to what you do or do not wish to retain from a teaching.

Throughout this book, you will find certain sentences placed inside a frame. These are intended to encourage the reader to stop and reflect. May I suggest you read these sentences three times, check how you feel when you read them, and allow them to sink in. Then, to truly KNOW if their import is good for you, you must try out these suggestions several times.

After all, a belief should only be accepted if it brings you a sense of wellbeing and a better quality of life, and not for any other reason. Every belief you decide to hold must therefore be one that is intelligent for you. Let me remind you, furthermore, that all beliefs are temporary because something new could occur anytime, prompting you to change them.

BELIEVING is defined as HOLDING something TO BE TRUE. But what is true for oneself at a given moment is not necessarily true for the rest of one's life. For instance, it may be true that it is not a good idea for a child of five to speak to a stranger on the street. However, if, as an adult, a person continues to see that childhood advice as a good idea for them, it could cause them serious problems.

The approach suggested in this book is totally complementary to any other approach that a person with cancer may have chosen, as it is principally metaphysical in nature and, above all, spiritual. It is my intention to help you find inner peace through a discovery of the hidden face of cancer.

This book is for anyone who is suffering from cancer or accompanying someone suffering from it or who is afraid of it because they know that there have been numerous cases in their family. It is also and especially for those who wish to find ways to protect themselves against it. In fact the main purpose of this book is first and foremost to prevent cancer. When you read the statistics appearing in the first chapter, you will see why improving them is long overdue.

My second goal is to help you stop seeing cancer as a burden, an ENEMY one has to fight at all costs or to which one must resign oneself in powerlessness. I want to help you become aware of just how much cancer can become a FRIEND, basically wanting to give you a message of hope, a way to recover inner peace.

I want to mention that I realize this book may be read by people who have never read any of my other books or taken any of the *Listen to Your Body* workshops. That is why you will find certain concepts of my teaching explained in detail, even though it may seem repetitive to those of you who are already familiar with them.

The colours used for the cover of this book were selected, as they are for all my books, on the basis of its content. Indeed, everything alive on this planet has a colour and every colour reflects something in particular while at the same time automatically influencing whatever it touches.

The colour pink eases tensions, brings gentle revitalization and exercises a positive influence on the body and the mind. In fact, it is the first colour to make us aware of the need to lessen the weight of bad memories. Chromotherapy also teaches that the colour pink has properties that heal the body and the mind and are capable of raising the body's vibration levels.

The colour turquoise for its part is a blend of blue and green, eliciting a purifying and balancing action from the green and a calming action from the blue. Turquoise also stimulates the immune system and fosters regeneration which aids healing. This colour furthermore brings a lot of hope and self-confidence.

As well, I always use purple for the print in my books. This colour allows you to read with your feelings rather than with your mind, which we tend to do when reading black print.

THE ORIGIN OF THE WORD CANCER

**It is to the great physician HIPPOCRATES – considered as the father of medicine – that we owe the derivation of this word. He used the words *carcinos* and carcinoma to describe two kinds of tumors. In Greek, these words refer to the crab. The way this illness develops made him think of the shape of a crab.**

**Four hundred years after him, the Roman physician CELSUS translated the Greek term into Latin, resulting in the word *cancer*.**

**About a century later, another Roman physician named GALEN used the Latin word *oncos* to describe a tumor and this word is still recognizable today as the root of the words *oncology* (the area of medicine that deals with cancer) and *oncologist* (a cancer specialist).**

# Chapter One

## Some interesting statistics

There are countless statistics about cancer available on the internet, from just about every country in the world. In this chapter I will present some of them, mainly in order to give you a more global picture of how widespread this illness is. You will be able to note, among other things, that approximately one in every four people who have cancer die from it. On the other hand, when a doctor makes the statement, you have a malignant tumor, he is not necessarily thereby saying, *YOU ARE DYING.* Why not decide to be part of the three out of four who survive?

It is true that we hear more and more talk about this illness today. Before, people didn't dare speak so openly about it. But the fear is still there and it's not hard to understand why. My hairstylist told me recently that twenty years ago she would hear the word "cancer" mentioned in her salon about once a week. Now, it's several times a day. Whether in relation to oneself or a loved one, cancer has become a very common subject of conversation, not just at the beauty salon, but everywhere, in personal as well as professional environments.

I have worked with many doctors since the founding of my school and most of them agree with me, telling me that this illness is increasingly the first thing they think of when a patient comes to see them about a new problem, especially if the problem is persistent. Quite often they fear it is cancer before they have even obtained the lab analysis results. As they are regularly confronted with this illness, one can hardly blame them.

For information purposes, here are the *Canadian Cancer Society's* statistics for 2012:

- 186,400 new cases of cancer (not including the 81,300 cases of skin cancer other than melanoma);
- 75,700 cases of death caused by this illness;
- More than 50% of these cases were lung cancer, colorectal (colon-rectum) cancer, prostate cancer or breast cancer;
- More than a quarter (27%) of all deaths due to cancer are attributable to lung cancer;
- 12% of all deaths are attributable to colorectal cancer;
- 69% of new cases of cancer and 62% of deaths from cancer affect people between 50 and 79 years of age;
- Between the ages of 20 and 50, the cancer rate is higher for women;
- Before 20 and after 50, the rate is higher for men.

Of 35,000,000 Canadians in 2012, 17,400,000 were men and 17,600,000 were women. Below are the statistics giving the number of new cases and the number of deaths for certain cancers for Canadian men and women in 2012. Note that only the six most common cancers have been cited and therefore the percentage of death is actually higher than that given above.

Among MEN, there were 97,600 new cases of cancer and a total of 39,500 deaths, that is, about 40%.

| | New cases | Deaths |
|---|---|---|
| Lung | 13,300 | 10,800 |
| Colorectal | 13,300 | 5,000 |
| Prostate | 26,500 | 4,000 |
| Pancreatic | 2,200 | 2,100 |
| Leukemia | 3,200 | 3,500 |
| Stomach | 2,100 | 1,350 |

Among Canadian WOMEN, there were 88,800 new cases of cancer and a total of 36,200 deaths, with the same percentage of deaths as the men, about 40%:

| | New cases | Deaths |
|---|---|---|
| Lung | 12,300 | 9,400 |
| Breast | 22,700 | 5,100 |
| Colorectal | 10,300 | 4,200 |
| Pancreatic | 2,300 | 2,100 |
| Ovarian | 2,600 | 1,750 |
| Uterine | 5,300 | 900 |

Most of the talk among men is about prostate cancer; eventually they learn that this cancer has the smallest percentage of deaths compared to the number of cases discovered. In 2012 in Canada, 73 new cases of prostate cancer were diagnosed each day, while there were 11 deaths from it each day.

It is a very similar situation for women with breast cancer. There is a lot of talk about it even though it is the one with the lowest percentage of deaths. Each day, 62 Canadian women learn that they have breast cancer while about 14 die from it each day.

This decrease in mortality is attributable mainly to cancer screening programs which help to detect new cases sooner.

On the whole, the incidence rates (new cases) are stable for men and increasing slightly for women. The good news is that the mortality rate is decreasing, which indicates that the survival rate for certain cancers is increasing.

I have only presented here the statistics for Canada, as they probably do not differ greatly from those of other developed countries. If, however, you want more information for another country, you will certainly be able to find it through a little internet research.

Most people hope that science will one day find a solution to cancer. For forty years, several health network sources have been telling us that in a few years there will be a solution they can offer us. Alas, this is not the case. Even if improvement has been achieved for some, the number of cancer cases has not ceased to increase over these last forty years. What is also unfortunate is that those who have undergone treatment and survived, but without obtaining the results they had hoped for, often have to accept several harmful side effects, such as healthy cells being attacked at the same time as the cancer cells, or the ablation of certain parts of the body.

In my internet research on statistics, I also learned that side effects from prescribed medications apparently constitute one of the leading causes of death. Likewise, we know that billions of dollars are spent each year to purchase medication, and the figure increases annually. That brings to mind what I saw on a visit to a nearby hospital last year when my husband was a patient there. How surprised I was that all the hospital corridors were lined with long tables piled high with towels, hospital gowns and other items that should have been stored in cupboards. There was barely enough room to get by.

When I asked a nurse what the justification was for this traffic congestion, she replied that for the last twenty years, the quantities of medication had increased so dramatically that they were taking up all the space in the cupboards formerly used for hospital room supplies. She furthermore confided to me that in those days, they had only one medication for dealing with any given condition while today there might be twenty or thirty.

I am well aware that progress in the field of pharmaceuticals has made it possible to bring patients relief and I am very happy these medications exist and are available when needed.

On the other hand, each of us has a duty to be more discerning and very vigilant regarding consequences. It is extremely important that you become informed about all the side effects of any long-term medication prescribed for you. Doctors may even suggest that you make a copy of this information for yourself, if you wish. However, keep in mind that most of them will not suggest this because the fear of side effects can at times do more harm than the illness itself. In any event, you can find all this information on the Internet.

All this to say that we must not rely only and entirely on medication to solve everything. The best approach is to have access to the type of medicine that we choose and to follow our intuition, but at the same time to look beyond the physical. We shall see in the chapters that follow how each of us can help reduce this mortality rate further by healing ourselves and especially by preventing the appearance of cancer in the first place.

All the statistics presented above are based, primarily, on the physical illness itself, as diagnosed and treated by conventional medicine. What I really wish to lead you to discover, dear reader, is how to look at this illness through new eyes and see it as a way to learn and a way to grow. It can help you become more conscious of marvellous and hidden aspects of yourself seeking to emerge through cancer. Seeing it this way, you will be able to help change and improve the statistics, which are actually just the temporary reflection of a small part of the population, as shown at the particular time a study was done.

Over the last thirty-plus years, I witnessed thousands of people who healed themselves by discovering that their ways of thinking were preventing them from truly loving themselves, and therefore from loving others unconditionally. I have had enough proof in recent years to convince me that behind all these illnesses, even if they are considered terminal and incurable, there exists a cause that goes well beyond the physical. I am not saying that everyone one I accompanied was healed, but at least they made significant progress spiritually, even if their body no longer had the strength or capacity to recover its natural state.

It is important you should be aware that well before I started developing and offering my teaching, I was already asking myself the following questions:

- Why does someone in good health, who eats properly, who doesn't drink or smoke and exercises everyday get cancer?

- Why does one person who is afraid of cancer attract it while another person who is afraid of it does not (the latter being the case of my mother)?

- Why do some people who smoke like a chimney never get cancer while it has been proven that tobacco is the leading cause of lung cancer?

- Why does a person who is fighting a cancer that has spread throughout her body and who is sent home with three months to live (like one of my aunts), die forty years later from a heart problem?

- Why is there always more cancer, when science seems to be making a lot of progress?

And how about you? What questions are you asking yourself? Perhaps the same ones I ask... and many others as well. If you have decided to read this book, it is because you surely have questions that are still unanswered, even if you are not conscious of them for the time being.

Now that I have had the good fortune of discovering the answers to all of these questions, I am keen to share them with you in this book. And it is my hope that they will be of as much help to you as they have been to me.

# Chapter Two

## The scientific and metaphysical explanation of cancer

Before explaining the connection between the scientific and metaphysical aspects of cancer, I need to describe briefly how I arrived at it. I became aware of the connection between our body and the way we think and live well before I founded my school. It was when the physical problems I had been suffering from for several years disappeared one after the other. This was possible only after I modified the way I was living, thanks to realizations that came to me from observing my dietary patterns. All the details are provided in my book *Just Listen to Your Body and Eat: Stop Trying to Control Your Weight.*

During the fifteen years prior, I had discovered the power of positive thinking to free me from several problems, including serious back pain, through visualization and programming. Each time, however, the remission would be only temporary, because using positive thinking is a method used to target one specific thing. So, I was constantly starting over. That's how I discovered that there was something else much deeper that was hiding behind all physical ailments. It was the beginning of my spiritual journey.

Taking a physical aspect and connecting it with a psychological aspect is called *metaphysics*. I enjoyed discovering that everything physical corresponded to something metaphysical. To be able to accept the idea that there is always an aspect beyond the physical, one must welcome the idea that the physical world is but a reflection of all that is happening on the mental and emotional levels. But we need especially to accept that illness, or any unpleasant situation arising in our life, may be compared to the tip of an iceberg coming into view. That tip is in fact hiding something much bigger and much more important.

**The more serious the illness or problem you are experiencing, the more likely the hidden part of the iceberg is massive.**

This ability to see the metaphysical aspect led me very quickly to see the spiritual aspect existing within all messages. In other words, when any ailment is discovered, we may be sure it is an indication of a lack of self-love, a lack that prevents us from listening to what our soul truly needs.

In reality each of us is a spiritual being, which I like to visualize as a resplendent ball of light. And this is true for everything that lives, whether mineral, plant, animal or human. This light wears a material envelope so as to be able to live on this planet. Were we to find ourselves on another planet, we would not be able to see the life animating it, because the nature of life over there would be particular to that planet. It would be bizarre, and even inconceivable, to believe that Earth is the only planet where there is life.

Our material envelope consists of three bodies: mental, emotional and physical. The mental and emotional bodies represent the psychological aspect of our life. If we start with the premise that the physical body is merely a reflection of what happens on the psychological level, it makes it easier to establish the connections between the physical and psychological aspects of the human.

Your inner light therefore represents your spiritual aspect, which I often call our inner GOD. It is that part of you that knows exactly what you need, but which also knows the reason why you have returned to this planet, that is, it knows the overall plan for your soul in this life.

Your inner GOD wants only your happiness in every sense of the word, and this is true for each one of us. If we got into the good habit of always following our intuition, and thus of listening to what our inner GOD tells us, everything would go perfectly smoothly in our life.

**Following the path of GOD means being in your heart, loving yourself, allowing yourself to be what you are, all the time.**

Over the centuries and the incarnations, we have unfortunately forgotten our inner GOD and consequently believe that we are our three bodies. These bodies have ended up usurping most of the space. In the natural order of things, they should always be at the service of our inner GOD, but, in reality, this is not what happens. Our bodies have progressively become our gods and we let them control us.

Your mental body is the one that helps you to think, memorize and organize, while it is your emotional body that allows you to have desires and feelings. Then there is your physical body which lets you move into action.

Take the example of a young man who, on a deep inner level, has always sensed the need to become an artist. He loves to paint. This expressed need comes from his inner GOD. To satisfy this need, he must use the capabilities of his three bodies. To ensure that he remains focused on what he wants, he must put himself in a situation "as if" all the circumstances were perfect and "as if" his decision would not upset anyone. Mentally, he must begin to visualize what would be required of him: which study programs to undertake, for how long, what this would cost, and so forth.

Throughout the planning stage, he will stay in touch with how he feels at the idea of carrying out his project. If he is assailed by doubts, he must quickly reconnect with the goal he set for himself. He will then have only to act on his plan.

Finally then, it is not how long it will take him to reach his goals that matters, but rather the happiness he will feel the closer he gets to reaching them. It is even very possible that he will have to find another job in order to meet his needs during the time it will take to complete his studies. Along the way, he will, on the other hand, experience many happy moments, just picturing that he will get there one day, as long as he does not lose sight of his objective.

Unfortunately, this is not how it goes in most cases. More likely, this young man will let himself be convinced by his friends and family that it is not very realistic to go into this kind of field, that he will never manage to make a career of it and, above all, that it will be almost impossible for him to make a decent living at it. They will try to convince him that he would be much smarter to choose an area like business, which his father worked in all his life.

If in the end he does succumb to the influence of his friends and family (who are a reflection of what is going on inside him), it is an indication that he believes the same thing they do. His fears will surely win out and he will probably follow their advice. What he does not realize is that he will never be happy with his decision, he will reject himself and hate himself for it for the rest of his life, even if he is not conscious of this. And it is this feeling of resentment, powerlessness, dissatisfaction with oneself and even hatred, which without question ends up causing illnesses of all sorts, possibly including cancer.

## The usefulness of illness

Illness, then, is a call from our inner GOD to recognize our inner power. It is a reminder that when we ignore this power, we show a lack of self-love. And this is when, one way or another, we will try to fill this void with all kinds of things or substances from our physical world.

**The more serious the illness, the more urgent the message from our inner GOD.**

**It is our soul crying *HELP*, for it knows full well that we are not living out our life plan in keeping with our needs.**

Any illness or problem arising in our life is always the last resort our GOD will use to draw our attention to a way of thinking that is hurting us as much as the illness or problem is. This implies that several other warnings were sent to us earlier, psychological as well as physical ones, but that we turned a deaf ear.

It is as if our GOD, who wants only a marvellous life for us, was asking us, *When are you going to catch on that it is high time for you to change the way you live, to make new decisions, to realize that what you are deciding to be at this moment is leading you directly away from the life you need and deserve?*

**Illness is always an indication that our life is being directed by our EGO instead of by our heart.**

The ego is created from mental and emotional energy, that is, from several memories filled with an emotional charge based on fear. These memories have become so important over time that they now direct our life. These harmful beliefs distance us from what our heart needs. I will describe in greater detail what is really meant by the word "ego" in the next chapter.

Our inner GOD is so desirous of our happiness that it draws to us everything we need to return to the light, even when it is not what we want. Carl Gustav Jung, the great psychoanalyst who did a vast amount of research on synchronicity, stated that we are part of a great whole, called the collective consciousness. We constantly attract to ourselves the people and situations we need in order to become conscious of those aspects of ourselves that we still find hard to accept.

I often use the word UNIVERSE to refer to this collective consciousness. In fact, there is no such thing as chance or coincidence: it is rather the Universe that is at work. I also like the way Einstein describes the word chance: chance is the name GOD goes by when GOD does not want to be recognized.

Let me return to the example of the young man I mentioned earlier. His soul was thus drawn intuitively to a family holding the same beliefs as he did. The close friends and family who influenced him not to listen to his need to be an artist certainly did not do this because they did not love him. Actually, they were quite simply led by their ego, their beliefs. The young man, through his inner GOD, attracted this experience in order to become aware of his own fears, which may have been directing him over several lifetimes. It is therefore an opportunity for him to become aware of a certain part of his life plan, to see that he is on this Earth with this type of family in order to recover mastery over his own life. He can then give himself permission to love himself sufficiently to attend to his need.

If instead he continues to go against his true need, it is very likely that he will end up attracting an illness, which will then help him to become conscious of the psychological harm he experiences following decisions made on the basis of fear rather than love.

**The pain and harmful consequences of an illness are always of the same intensity as the pain experienced by the soul when its needs are not being attended to.**

Some people believe in fate, claiming that if they are to die of cancer or of something else, it is simply their destiny being played out. Why not, on the other hand, decide to believe that we create our destiny ourselves along the way throughout our lives, attracting to ourselves everything that we need in order to live consciously? Thus, the more conscious we become, the greater our opportunity to create the destiny we desire.

Others believe that illnesses are due to genetic predisposition or heredity and that it is normal to have the same pathologies as our biological parents. This has been a common belief for a long time and it was held by physicians as well. But the medical profession has gradually come to realize that many illnesses once considered to be "hereditary" can no longer be viewed that way.

Based on a study of a large number of adopted children, a group of researchers discovered that they had a five times greater risk of having cancer if one of the two ADOPTIVE parents had it. This confirms that children do not necessarily inherit cancer from one of their parents, but they could develop the same illnesses only if they decide to continue to hold certain beliefs inspired by their parents, biological or not.

## Changing our DNA

Ever since scientists have been studying people's DNA, they constantly discover new things. For example, there have been studies of identical twins, who would of course have been born with identical DNA, which showed that they developed different illnesses and sometimes died at different ages, even as many as ten years apart. They had no option but to confirm that DNA changed over time, according to people's behaviours and attitudes.

Quantum physics also reached this conclusion, proving that our consciousness models our world. Researchers have furthermore observed electrons which, once they became solid, behaved like waves in their normal state in accordance with the intention of the person doing the observing. One thing led to another and they realized that our DNA could be changed by our intentions. It is in fact our intentions that help us to take different decisions, which in my opinion, is the determining factor for changing DNA.

Another thing I have learned is that if we were to adopt a new behaviour or a new attitude and put it into practice for at least three months, a new connection between two neurons in our brain would be created. In fact, the brain is capable of holding up to several billion neurons connected to one another. These are the same connections that make us behave in a habitual manner, that represent our beliefs and make us act systematically in the same way. For example, when you receive criticism, your initial reaction might be one of anger whereas for someone else it might be to clam up.

I would like to offer a metaphysical explanation with regard to DNA. Is it possible that this new connection is created at the same time as a change in our DNA? As I write this, I think of, among others, Norman Cousins, the American who learned that his cancer had spread and that he had only three months to live. After his discharge from hospital, he rented tons of comedy movies and bought humorous books. He only allowed people who could make him laugh to visit him. He very quickly noted that after fifteen minutes of laughter, he would not feel any pain for two hours and that he could rest without taking any pain medication.

After a few months, he was pronounced cured. He then undertook the writing of a book entitled *Anatomy of an Illness as Perceived by the Patient: reflections on healing and regeneration* and went on to specialize in teaching about healing through laughter. It is thanks to him moreover that laughter therapy got its start. It is now used all over the world. Cousins was the first American to be appointed professor of medicine while not a medical doctor.

THIS MAN CHANGED HIS DNA. There you have the answer to a question I posed in Chapter One concerning one of my aunts who also healed herself by making a new decision. The form of our DNA is the expression of our genes and, as I understand it, our genes are the expression of our beliefs – on the physical, emotional and mental levels.

**That is why we are not prisoners of the genetic baggage with which we enter the world at birth.**

Your soul was drawn to a family having the same beliefs as you and the same issues to deal with. That is why they say, in medicine and in psychology, that if one parent has cancer, depression or suicidal tendencies..., there is a strong chance that you will have the same thing. I agree with this statement but only if the child does not change anything in their attitude and makes no effort to accomplish their life plan. Everyone's life plan is one of transformation and ceasing to believe in anything that separates us from love of self and others. That is why it is rightly said that each new generation outshines the last. This is not a reference to physical progress, but to progress in the realm of the soul and the ability to love.

**Your DNA therefore does not control you, any more than your three bodies do, which must be at the service of your greater self, your spiritual self, your inner GOD.**

In summary, the metaphysical helps you make the connection between what is happening in your physical body and what is happening beyond the physical level.

## Hidden behind the scientific aspect

When we read the scientific definition of cancer or a detailed description of it, we learn a lot about those who suffer from it. What follows is my metaphysical interpretation, based on that description:

| Scientific | Metaphysical |
|---|---|
| Cancer begins when a cell in our body attacks us. | The cancerous cell corresponds to a part of our ego that considers us guilty enough to justify attack. |
| Cancer does not come from outside of us, as happens with a bacterial infection, for example. | We are attacking ourselves. It is not someone else who is attacking us. |
| The cell is no longer behaving in accordance with its natural function or its DNA coding. It multiplies incessantly, taking up more and more space, destroying everything in its path. | There is a harmful belief that is not following the divine laws of Love. It completely invades the person, in all spheres of their life. |
| The cancerous cell regresses and seems to want to behave like the first cell formed by the mother's ovum and the father's sperm, which are meant to divide and multiply to form a complete being. | This part of us, this harmful belief, seeks to go backwards, tries to reconstruct itself and start over in order to take up more space. It does not realize it is destroying and not building anything new. |

| | |
|---|---|
| A normal adult cell knows its limits. For example, the cells that multiply in order to heal a wound know they must stop when the two sides of the wound meet. The cancerous cell does not recognize its limits. | When we follow our heart, we can tell intuitively if we have reached our limit. But the suffering part in us goes beyond its limits of suffering, and has therefore lost control. It is taking up far too much space in our life. |
| When a cancer reappears, the cells are considered to have developed resistance and the cancer is said to be more virulent, like bacteria that develop resistance to antibiotics, requiring stronger antibiotics to constantly be developed. The same applies to drugs for pain control. | When we have not wanted to grasp the message the first time, because of the resistance of our ego, the ego returns to the offensive all the more forcefully, in the hope of regaining control over our life. |
| It is also said that every person produces cancerous cells (cells that are prone to multiply too fast or altered cells) at various times in their life, but that a healthy immune system recognizes them right away and destroys them. In the case of cancer, the harmful cells are stronger than the immune system. | The *thymus* plays an important role in protecting against auto-immunity. This organ is directly related to the heart chakra (the chakra representing self-love). This tells us that an immune system that is too weak to do its work properly is a reflection of a person significantly weakened by their lack of self-love and whose self-hate is stronger than their self-love. |

| | |
|---|---|
| It has been observed that cancer is sometimes preceded by chronic inflammations. | In metaphysics, inflammation is a sign of of anger. The more there is repressed anger present, the greater the possibility of cancer. |
| Another known fact is that adrenalin nourishes cancer cells, prompting them to develop more rapidly. | Adrenalin is the hormone released into our system to help us face fear. We can deduce from this that the more a person is afraid, the faster the cancer cells in their body will develop. This explains why certain cancers are more virulent than others. |

I also want to share with you some interesting research on the immune system. I heard about this research several years ago and it was carried out at an American university specializing in paranormal phenomena, using a group of students as the subject. The directors of the research tested each student's immune system before they invited them to watch two films.

Examination of the students' immune systems after they had viewed the first film, which contained violence, revealed that in most cases, the system had been significantly weakened. The second film was about Mother Teresa caring for lepers and taking them into her arms to comfort them and give them love. Unaccustomed to this type of film, several of the students appeared uncomfortable but they had to watch the film to the end. At the second examination of the immune system, after the second film, the doctors observed in every case that the system had become stronger.

From this they concluded that love and serenity strengthen the immune system, helping it accomplish what it needs to do, while violence, hate and anger weaken it, making us less resistant to anything that might attack us.

In the chapters that follow, further information and several other explanations will be added to what is provided in the chart above.

A link between cancer and repressed emotions has now been established for a very long time. The first time I myself heard of it was in the 70s, when I was attending personal growth workshops in schools in the U.S. Cancer was defined as an emotional sickness.

As early as the start of the last century, many psychiatrists, the first being Sigmund Freud, followed by his student Wilhelm Reich and then Carl Gustav Jung, made the link between the health problems people experience and their psychological state. Jung said, *What we do not want to acknowledge in ourselves will invariably manifest itself in our body.* Even Hippocrates, the father of medicine, the great Greek doctor who lived some 1600 years ago, stated that it was the black bile humour – melancholy and sadness – that was hiding behind cancer. He looked at four different humours and confirmed that there was a link between a person's temperament and the various illnesses that might derive from it.

In most countries, an increasing number of doctors are writing on this subject and they have been doing so for at least fifty years. Among them is the renowned Dr. Carl Simonton who was one of its great pioneers. Each of them presents a very interesting and slightly different understanding of this phenomenon and I encourage you to read their books to broaden your horizons.

We are always delighted when a new participant tells us it was their doctor who suggested they come and take a workshop with us at our school in order to better understand the meaning of their illness. Not a week goes by without this happening in all the countries where we teach. I consider all these doctors to be real physicians of the body and of the soul.

When a client tells us they no longer have confidence in traditional medicine and that they refuse to go and see their doctor, we strongly suggest that they look for a doctor with an open mind, or seek out alternative medicine options. What matters most is that while someone else is providing physical care, they help themselves by doing the inner work to which they are being called by their illness. Be aware that medicine, metaphysics and spirituality can all work together.

I am certain that in the years ahead fewer and fewer doctors and therapists will try to convince their patients that their approach is the only way to deal with their symptoms or cure them. In the past, I even encountered workshop facilitators – associated with certain schools – who were so sure they held the only truth for everyone that they forbade people to use their methods without obtaining permission.

Those who revel in this kind of attitude are unfortunately using their methods to prove to themselves that they exist. I dream of the day when all health care professionals will have only the wellbeing of their patients at heart, achieved by whatever means is most effective. We all know already that there are numerous ways of addressing GOD and connecting with

GOD in this world. There are likewise several ways to deal with illness. What matters is what the person who is ill ultimately decides.

**You are the only one with the power to choose what type of medicine will suit you best. Use this power, then, out of love for yourself.**

It is your body and your life. Therefore you are the only person who can assume the consequences of your decisions. Remember that you must have confidence in the person attending to you. If you do not, your chances of healing will be significantly reduced. You can also choose to receive help from multiple disciplines at the same time, each of them having something to offer you, as long as it is your choice.

This makes me think of all the people who have asked me, over these last thirty years, who my master or guru is. Personally, I have never wanted to follow the teachings of just one person. In the last forty-five years, I have taken part in a great many workshops and read countless books and I have always been able to learn something new from each of them.

The more you are open to the intelligence and knowledge of others, the more you will be in a position to develop your own. Throughout all these years, I had managed without realizing it, to develop a great ability to synthesize everything I absorbed from others. Without warning, an idea comes to me, and strikes me as particularly right and true. In fact, these moments of inspiration are always a great source of joy for me and they are extremely energizing.

The same is true of medicine. The more a doctor or therapist is interested in a variety of disciplines, the greater their capacity for synthesis and the more tools they have available for helping their patients. They will know intuitively what is needed in each case. I am fortunate to know a good many such doctors, whom I would be glad to recommend. If all doctors and therapists could convince their patients that they and only they have the power to truly heal themselves, I am absolutely convinced that far more people would experience healing.

## The importance of intelligence

Along the same lines, I dare to hope that one day we will find people of great wisdom like those we had in ancient times, who can synthesize everything that specialists have been able to discover. During the last fifty years, science keeps turning out specialists in every field, each holding their truth, often in contradiction with one another, it seems. When I speak of people of great wisdom in former times, individuals like Leonardo da Vinci come immediately to mind. He was at the same time an artist, scientist, engineer, inventor, anatomist, painter, sculptor, architect, urbanist, botanist, musician, philosopher and writer. Not bad for a single human being!

I sincerely believe that a wholistic vision is possible, for we are entering the Age of Aquarius. It will be a great era for the development of intelligence and global vision in all fields. We are already feeling the energy of Aquarius (the Water carrier), especially since the sixties. Indeed, there are great transformations taking place on our planet and there is a growing trend toward people wanting to be informed.

It will be a highly spiritual era, thanks to which we will receive increased energy to help us accept who we are, to help us accept *being what we are, all of the time*, rather than constantly seeking *to have* and *to do.*

**We are not human "haves" or «do's", we are human BEINGS.**

This means then that the material dimension must be at the service of the spiritual dimension. Furthermore, everything is being accelerated – including time – with this new energy. We are receiving much from beyond, unbeknownst to us, in order to increase our inner power. Unfortunately, many people misuse their power, that is to say, they create what they do not want rather than what they want.

## What is the difference between intelligence and intellect?

An *intelligent* person is one who seeks to find solutions that will meet their general needs, one who seeks therefore what is beneficial and who is always conscious of the law of cause and effect. This kind of person does not want to invent or use as a solution something that may have a harmful effect on them, on those around them or on their environment.

An *intellectual* person is one who seeks to acquire knowledge and has a great capacity for memorization. For this person, the possession of knowledge is more important than feeling or experience.

I discovered this difference when I worked in sales. I realized that if a representative knew their product very well but was more concerned about not forgetting any details and doing a perfect presentation, he or she did not have much success in sales. On the other hand, if the representative was convinced of the benefits of the product and made sure it would benefit the client (thereby making it an intelligent purchase for the client), he or she was much more successful, even if they sometimes forgot certain details about the product. The client experienced the presentation in a more positive way. Only after several years of working in this field did I finally understand the reason for my success: I functioned in the latter way and did so intuitively without having learned it from anyone.

The ideal is to be as intellectual as we are intelligent, while at the same time keeping in mind that our intellect must always be at the service of our intelligence. When you see a person who is able to remember, for instance, every detail about their product and can at the same time share what they feel about its benefits, you are getting a good picture of a person who is using both their intellect and their intelligence.

I am bold enough to hope that there will be an increasing number of doctors and therapists who are qualified not only by virtue of their knowledge but by virtue of their intelligence as well. By intelligence here I mean the ability to listen and show compassion toward their patients. This brings to mind, among other things, an incident I experienced when I was an adolescent at convent school with the nuns. As part of an examination in *Composition,* we were to write a story of at least 10 pages. Believe it or not, this was the subject that interested me the least at the time. When I learned I had received a much higher mark than my friend because I hadn't made any spelling errors, I felt it to be very unfair and not very intelligent. In my view, it wasn't a grammar exam, but a composition exam. My friend wrote so much better than I did, with great imagination and poetry, but unfortunately, she had no talent for grammar.

Happily, times have changed. I have been able to observe, over my thirty-one years of teaching the *Listen to Your Body* philosophy in more than twenty-two countries, that a broadening of consciousness and of intelligence is taking place just about everywhere. The era we live in is thus marked by a great revolution in consciousness and is proving to be a more intelligent one which cannot fail to simultaneously engender a great scientific revolution. The emergence of *quantum physics* has moreover shown this to be true. It has thrown into question a whole series of theories and beliefs previously held by the scientific world.

Ever since DNA was discovered, genetic research has also led to many questions that still remain unanswered. For example, we now know that a monkey has 99% of the same genes as a human. The greatest difference noted in the human is their consciousness, their intelligence, their ability to make great discoveries, etc. But to this day, scientists have been unable to find any genes to match those criteria.

What good news! Finally, we have discovered that the human is endowed with more than a physical body and that human intelligence is located somewhere other than inside it.

# Chapter Three

## The influence of the wound of rejection

I mentioned earlier that several researchers and authors offer very interesting and different interpretations on the basis of their particular research and observations. Likewise, I offer mine. I agree that repressed emotions have a direct influence on cancer, but my approach focuses specifically on associating those emotions with the wound of *REJECTION.*

For the past twenty years I have been explaining my wounds theory which I will now share with you. You will find a great many answers here to all sorts of problems that every one of us experiences.

One of the teachings of this theory is that we are all born with soul wounds and they are five in number: *rejection, abandonment, humiliation, betrayal and injustice.* From my observations over all these years, I have concluded that we are all born with at least four of the five wounds, humiliation being the only one not common to everyone.

It is important to know that these wounds are generally experienced in different degrees. Most people are affected by at least two major wounds, which are likewise activated more or less often and with varying frequency and intensity, depending on the situations they are in and the people involved.

Every wound is awakened by our parents – or by those who have played a parental role – between the time of our birth and the age of seven (I use the word *awakened* because the wound is already inscribed in our soul before birth). In fact, psychological research has shown that we have already experienced all the emotions we will experience throughout the rest of our life during our first seven years on this planet, and have also developed the sum total of our beliefs by that time. After the age of seven, there is only repetition to help make us conscious of what we as an individual do or do not accept.

Alas, consciousness is not awakened fast enough. Many people in their sixties still live the same emotions they did when they were six with their parents or other family members. Some may have become more aware of the emotions they experience, but take no new decisions that could help them live with greater inner peace. Many schools of thought concur that, on average, people are conscious of less than 10% of what is going on inside them. Fortunately, the new era we are entering constantly offers us myriad ways to awaken consciousness. This leads me to believe that we shall make great strides of progress in this regard in the years to come.

In my book about our wounds[1], I offer a detailed explanation of each of the five wounds, including how to recognize them in our physical body, the different attitude for each wound when it is activated, how to heal the wounds and the beneficial transformation in a person the more these wounds are healed. In the present book, I will focus only on the wound of rejection which in my view is the wound that, when it becomes too activated, is at the root of repressed emotions. And repressed emotions are a significant cause of cancer.

## Resistance and discernment

You may feel resistance in yourself as you read what I have just said or what I am about to write. I suggest, however, that

1 *Heal your wounds and find your true self,* published by LES EDITIONS ETC.

you avoid fighting this resistance because it may be precisely the thing to help you develop discernment. Let me remind you that all the theories you have heard so far, as well as the innumerable other theories that will increasingly appear as our knowledge and consciousness continue to open up further, may not be what you need. In the final analysis, you must use your discernment and your intuition to decide what really works for you.

To make good decisions in this regard, it is recommended that you follow through with the theory, being attentive all the while to your feelings. If a new theory provides answers to your questions, or greater clarity and understanding in you, and contributes to your feeling better, you will then know that it works *for you for the time being*. If you experience doubts or feel some degree of discomfort when reading or listening to a new theory, make sure that it is coming from your intuition and not from fears based on what you have learned in the past, like the fears mentioned at the very start of this book.

## The ego and beliefs

All resistance is an indication that your ego has gotten the upper hand. What is the ego? In practical terms, it is the totality of your beliefs. It is therefore at the root of all your problems, both physical and psychological. But how could the human race have developed such an ego, which unfortunately directs most people's lives? To better grasp its importance, we need to accept the fact that the soul arrives with its baggage of countless lives. This explains how the ego grows from one life to the next for however long we allow it to do so and abdicate our power to it.

As soon as your thoughts settle on something bothering you, worrying you, or causing you to feel certain emotions or fears, it means that you are no longer centered and that your ego has taken over. Be aware that the ego is always built on what it has learned and has great difficulty being open to something new. When you are centered, there is no inner disquiet and you can dwell in the present moment.

For example, when an idea comes to you spontaneously, it is coming from your inner GOD and not your mental body. As soon as you question it and feel anxious about it, you know that your ego has taken over the idea. It questions every new idea that comes from someone else. Its mantra is, "If you don't think like me, if you believe in something other than me, you are less than me and you are wrong."

To remain in your present moment when you have a new idea or another person inspires you with one, simply make a mental note of it and see if it makes you go WOW. After that, you let the Universe do its work in you. All that remains for you to do after that is to have confidence in your inner GOD who will constantly guide you to know if, when, and how to pursue this idea.

It is your ego that clings to things, pleasures, people, suffering, etc. It is also your ego that incessantly wants to prove its superiority with those things it clings to. In this way it seeks to show you and everyone around you that it is so important that it can direct your life for you. What your ego doesn't know is that it has no idea what the needs of your inner being are, because the ego was created out of mental energy, memories and beliefs. Therefore it relies on these to determine whether or not something is good for you.

**A belief begins at a moment when we think we have hurt another person and, in this regard, feared greatly for ourselves.**

**We have decided that being and acting that way was bad and that we should not act that way again so that we will not experience that fear for ourselves again.**

IN OTHER WORDS, WE HAVE NOT ACCEPTED OUR SELF. It is the **decision** to *not be like this anymore* that starts to create the belief. Each time we act that way afterwards, or that we see someone else act this way toward us or with others, or that we behave this way toward ourselves, we judge it as BAD and add another layer of intensity to the belief and the fear.

We can become aware of a belief when another person acts a certain way toward us and it bothers us. This helps us realize that if we are receiving this from another person, it means we have already behaved this way toward ourselves and toward another person.

It is very important to remember that what we experience from others has to do with BEING and not on the basis of their behaviour. I will furthermore return to this point often throughout this book. So, when a behaviour disturbs us, we should immediately ask ourselves what we are judging this person to BE. Every judgment of a person, even in circumstances that do not concern you, indicate that you do not accept this attitude, because your ego believes it is bad to be this way.

Each of your beliefs is associated with one or more wounds. If the same belief awakens two wounds, it is a sign of very strong belief leading to very strong resistance and control in your life. The stronger this belief, the greater the tricks it can play on you and the more it can make you believe you are not like that, only others are. We can conclude from this that people with a reputation for having a big ego are simply people who suffer a lot because they have bigger and deeper wounds.

Take the example of the baby girl who refuses breastfeeding because she feels intuitively her mother is emotionally very upset. The mother, who was so much looking forward to this experience of nursing, is unhappy with the situation, chooses to bottle-feed her baby, and is not as affectionate as she could be. She surely does not realize that it is her wound of rejection that has just been activated by her baby's attitude.

Mommy feels rejected, just like the little girl does, and a vicious circle is set into motion. It will continue for as long as they both have not figured out how to love themselves. The little voice inside them that says, "I must really be no good and not very important if the person I love wants nothing to do with me," grows louder and louder as the belief gets stronger and stronger.

The greater the wounds, by virtue of having been activated in one life after another, the more beliefs there will be that correspond to each of these wounds. Accordingly, the ego's power can take on huge proportions. Humans have allowed their ego to dominate them for such a long time that they have entirely forgotten their divine power with all its potential for creating a happy life.

**Our ego thinks it is our god, for it is we who have created it and given it all our power.**

We have reached a crucial moment on this planet when we must absolutely take back our power and stop feeding our ego more energy. If we cease to nourish it, it will gradually diminish.

## When is the wound of rejection activated?

Your wound of rejection is activated as soon as you feel rejected by someone else, or you reject yourself or you believe you have rejected another person. This behaviour is so subtle that it is very difficult for most people to notice it right away.

Why is it so difficult? Because it is the wound that, out of the five, does the most harm and is the most sensitive. It is the only one that touches the deepest part of our BEING. This wound is already well awakened before birth, in the fetal stage, due to the various sounds, noises or conversations that the baby hears and feels coming from its mother and her surroundings. Let us take, for example, the case of one of the parents, or even both of them, not seeming to desire this child at the time. The baby may hear words like, *I hope at least it will be a boy and not a girl,* when the baby *is* a girl. Or, *Oh, no, not pregnant. It's really not the right time.*

Due to its wound of rejection, the baby receives such comments as a painful blow. It is convinced that the parent who made this kind of remark does not want it, while what they were really doing was expressing their limits at that moment or in the context of a personal problem.

**What most people take as rejection is in reality only the expression of certain limits by the other person.**

The wound of rejection is always awakened by the parent of the same sex or by the person who played the role of that parent at birth. Afterwards, it continues to be more and more activated, especially by people of the same sex as ourselves and at times by people of the opposite sex.

As soon as the baby starts feeling the pain of this wound, their first reaction is to try to escape into the realm of the soul, where they can convince themselves that all is well. This is why the larger the person's wound of rejection, the easier it will be to escape into their own world, an unreal world which they create for themselves.

Later on, people will say of them that they often *have their head in the clouds.* Some even create multiple personalities for themselves, a psychological problem in which the person doesn't remember what they are doing while they take on a secondary personality. Throughout our life, we use all sorts of means of escape in an effort to avoid suffering. Unfortunately, the suffering remains present all the same, but buried deep inside us.

Surely you are beginning to understand why this wound is the one that has the greatest potential for causing cancer to develop, as everything is kept inside. No longer being ourselves, it is as if we are wearing a mask so that no one will know what we feel or experience. Every wound possesses its own mask and every mask is recognizable by the behaviour of the person. The mask associated with the wound of rejection is called WITHDRAWER.

The behaviour and inner attitude of someone wearing the *withdrawer* mask is described below. Even if you are already familiar with the wounds, I wish to remind you of the characteristics of the *withdrawer,* as this will help you to make a clear connection between this attitude and cancer. I want to emphasize that all of the characteristics listed would be found in a person whose wound of rejection is major. Since each of our wounds has different degrees of intensity, it may be that some characteristics do not apply to you.

## Activation of the withdrawer mask

- The *withdrawer* is deeply convinced of being worthless or not worth much. They consider themselves a loser and without value. They have very little self-esteem. The greater the wound, the more worthless they feel in various fields and with different people;
- They are convinced that if they did not exist, it would not make much difference to those around them;
- They feel isolated and misunderstood;
- At a very early age, they became convinced that no one wanted to listen to them, the result being a withdrawal into self in adulthood. They feel they do not have the right to speak up;
- They are always on the lookout, observing everything and listening carefully to the words others use, often seeing reality in a distorted way and concluding that others are rejecting them;
- They usually say little and withdraw from a group. They are seen as solitary beings and people are inclined to want to leave them alone;
- The more their wound is repressed, the more their voice becomes inaudible;

- The more they isolate themselves, the more they seem to become invisible;
- They are specialists in denial, at making themselves believe that something doesn't bother them or that certain things didn't really happen;
- They will often claim everything is just fine for fear of bothering others or burdening them with their problems;
- As they are often in denial, they cannot feel or experience their physical and emotional limits;
- They are also inclined to want to deny what is happening to others and will tell them, *Don't worry, it doesn't matter, don't give it another thought;*
- They do not attribute much importance to material things: they are more attracted by matters pertaining to the invisible world and knowledge;
- They are not only perfectionists but great idealists who, as they age, feel more and more panic-stricken by the idea of not living up to their own expectations and those of others. They gradually develop an obsessive character;
- In their vocabulary they often use words like: *useless, nothing, disappear, non-existent, no room;*
- They refuse to feel their pain, minimize it to the maximum and just keep explaining it away;
- They believe that they are their beliefs and find it very difficult to become dissociated from them;

- They believe they are what they do: *If I do fine, then I am fine;*

- They are so lacking in love for themselves that they seek it from those around them, yet have a hard time accepting it because they believe they are too undeserving;

- They do not want to be like their parent of the same sex but feel lost or powerless at the thought of having no model to follow;

- They hate themselves as much as they hate the parent of the same sex;

- They may make themselves believe that it is the parent of the opposite sex that they hate the most, but when the latter is tough or rude with them, they hate the parent of the same sex even more for not coming to their defence and they feel rejected by that parent. In that case another one of the five wounds is activated with the parent of the opposite sex.

- Their greatest fear is PANIC.

It is very possible that you do not see yourself this way but be aware of denial. It can easily play tricks on you. In fact I suggest you check with those who are close to you, especially those who are not afraid to be honest with you, as to how they see you, perceive you, what characteristics they associate with you, and so forth. It is often easier for others to observe how much other people reject themselves. When we are in denial, we increasingly adopt another personality to make ourselves (and others) believe that we are not like this. We can have an air of self-confidence even when deep down, we may be terrified of inviting criticism. Denial is a commonly used means of running away from an unpleasant situation.

The *withdrawer* is convinced that using escape, which shows up in different forms, is the only way they can live without having to feel the pain of rejection because, when they feel that pain, it makes them panic. One might escape not only by running away physically from a situation, but also through sleep, medication, alcohol, drugs, tobacco, food, etc. This is why we often hear it said that smoking cigarettes, drinking alcohol or eating certain foods can cause cancer. I remember that when I was younger, the means of escape that I had found was shopping. I would go into a store and buy myself something I didn't really need, some small extravagance. When I got home, I felt good. What I had just done was put a lid on the feeling of fear that inhabited me at the time.

Let me reassure you, there are very few people who constantly display the attitudes and behaviours I have just described. It is only when your wound of rejection is activated, and you decide (unconsciously) to wear your *withdrawer mask,* that you manifest this kind of attitude. Often it is an automatic reaction to don this mask and thus adopt one or more of the behaviours described above.

**The more rejected we feel, the stronger and faster our reaction. Through this reaction, we create the illusion for ourselves that we can stop the suffering.**

As you can imagine, those who wear the *withdrawer* mask generally tend to prefer being alone. Finding it difficult to stay with their feelings for very long, they do not share them with others. The times when they tried to talk about them when they were younger, they felt their parents did not want to listen. This taught them to withdraw more and more over time. Through their ego, their wound convinced them that they were right to feel inferior.

If you have attracted this kind of behaviour from a parent, you need to realize it is your belief that you are inferior and that no one could be interested in what's happening with you that has attracted them in the first place. According to your parents, they were not rejecting you, they were just expressing their limits. Moreover, they were unconsciously a reflection of you.

Every event in your life, whether pleasant or unpleasant, is produced or develops in accordance with what is emanating from your deepest self. This can explain, among other things, why perhaps you did not choose the best time to speak to your parent, or maybe your parent was a bit awkward and did not use the right words to express himself or herself.

To achieve some kind of recognition, the *withdrawer* constantly seeks to BE more and more perfect, finally convincing themselves that only their good actions prove they exist. They are so afraid of not being perfect that they will inevitably attract the very object of their fear, make a mistake and end up feeling rejected all over again. What a vicious circle!

A young woman shared with me that when she was a child she used to hide behind a chair to see how long it would take the rest of the family to discover her absence. Sometimes she would wait several hours. It confirmed her belief that her existence mattered so little that no one realized she was missing.

The *withdrawer* is also a veritable specialist in distorting reality. Their over-active imagination continually plays tricks on them. Imagination is certainly one of the great gifts with which we humans have been endowed but unfortunately it is often used to imagine what we do not want instead of what we really need.

Have you ever made a mistake at work that inadvertently created a problem for certain people? You apologized and the people involved accepted your apology, saying that anyone can make a mistake. But if you keep thinking about it, calling yourself stupid, irresponsible, hopeless, not very bright, etc., then you are distorting reality because of your guilt feelings. The reality is probably that you were trying to do too many things at once and did not take care to re-check your work and did not mean to cause anyone a problem. Instead of apologizing, you would have done better to give yourself the right to be human – with strengths and weaknesses.

This kind of behaviour is a clear illustration of the obsessive character that develops in the *withdrawer* in proportion to the size of their wound of rejection. They will think endlessly about situations from the past or the future. It becomes difficult for them to be in the present moment and accept themselves as they are.

They are so self-deprecating that they constantly feel a great fear of being themselves and taking their rightful place. They are afraid that if they do, everyone will discover how inept they are. But when they don't stand up for themselves, it impossible for others to respect them. In fact, only THEY have the power to take the place to which they are naturally entitled. The *withdrawer* wants so much for others to give them a place that they cannot help but seek this by trying to be perfect, according to some idealistic image they have created.

But this image is simply not a realistic one. The *withdrawer* is a perfectionist-idealist who sets unattainable goals. It is interesting to note that the antonym of the word *ideal* is *real.* Hence, the more idealistic we are, the more unrealistic we become.

**Being a perfectionist can be very useful in itself, as long as we remain realistic and recognize our limits.**

The *withdrawer* suffers from a lack of love to the point of developing a hatred for their parent of the same sex as them who was unable to fill this void. As the soul is attracted by a parent of the same sex who will serve as a model, the child has a great dislike of this parent for not being a good model. Since they do not want to be like this parent, they find they have no model. They are very disappointed in this parent who does not know how to show them the love they crave, does not know how to acknowledge them and give them all the space they need. It is therefore normal and human that they should finally have no regard for this parent, for that is the person who, in most cases, will have occasioned our first big emotional pain.

As an infant, we do not have the emotional maturity needed to know that our parent of the same sex as us cannot give us or convey to us the love that we seek, because they too are suffering rejection. They too are failing to acknowledge themselves. They too lacked a parental model of the same sex that they could admire. Nor did they receive the love they craved from that parent. It continues thus from generation to generation, with the same sex, for as long as we are unable to develop self-love, that is, to accept who we are. I will come back to this topic in the final chapter.

## Link between the wounds of rejection and injustice

For most people, the further development of their wound of injustice starts around the age of four. This is to create a shell so they will feel the rejection even less. This wound gives the suffering person an additional tool for not feeling, the main tool they used earlier being escape. The mask this person develops with their wound of injustice is called *rigid.*

The wound of injustice is also awakened by the parent of the same sex. In fact, the two wounds are very often awakened during a single event or through the same person.

To know which wound is more affected in your case, observe your reaction carefully. If you are immediately outraged and express it verbally or with an action, it is your wound of injustice that is at work at that moment. How strongly and quickly you react reflects the degree of pain experienced. If on the other hand you choose to withdraw, to deny the situation or to say nothing, it is your wound of rejection that is being most affected at that instant.

An example of activated wounds comes to mind that happened to me recently at an airport. After receiving my boarding pass, I head toward the gate and am stopped at two different points where my pass and passport are checked. A bit farther along I see another representative of the airline checking another woman's passport. I walk past that agent because I tell myself it couldn't be yet a third checkpoint. I have gone only a few steps when the agent shouts at me, *Madame, you cannot go through, you must show me your passport. I'm NOT INVISIBLE, am I?*

Indeed, this agent presented a great many characteristics of the wound of rejection and injustice in her body. I could feel how much she must reject herself to express it even with people she did not know at her place of work. For her, the role of checking each person who goes through certainly gives her the feeling she is visible and that she exists. On the other hand, I am quite sure she is not aware of this fact and is convinced that she is doing a very good job. Certainly she can give the impression of having a big ego, of believing she is someone else, but in reality, she is just one among so many who suffer from a lack of self-love. Her remark indicates that her wound of injustice had the upper hand, speaking to me in that tone, just to keep her wound of rejection well hidden.

However, don't be fooled. Even if you notice that you are more often in your wound of injustice and that you wear the mask of *rigid,* it doesn't mean you never felt rejected. The pain of the rejection is simply buried, imprisoned behind your *rigid* shell which makes you behave differently. The suffering thus continues to build up inside you.

**It is when you reach your limit and you refuse to see it that the cancer may appear.**

It is as if you had been pulling on a big rope since the day you were born and it finally snapped. In every person suffering from cancer that I have worked with, I have observed that the two wounds of rejection and injustice were very much present. That is why the message in your physical body is so important. As I pointed out in the previous chapter, cancer does not originate outside of us, but rather comes from within. It is therefore initially activated by the wound of rejection and then by the wound of injustice which is subsequently superimposed on it.

The individual reaches their emotional limits and generates cells that lose control.

I want to clarify that when a person wears their *rigid* mask, they are aware that they are experiencing anger – which is not the case for the *withdrawer* – but they use a lot of control, since they believe it is not good to express their anger. Only a rigid person will manage to control their anger in this way. However, the people around them will recognize it easily enough when they see the tensing body, the tightening jaw and facial muscles. You can imagine then, and easily understand, that between the *withdrawer's* denial and the *rigid's* control, the person will end up reaching the limits of their endurance or "come to the end of their rope."

Let me remind you that even if the wound of rejection is not very apparent in a person, it is still very much there. What is happening is that the wound is so strongly denied that it turns up in disguise, tucked away under their other wounds.

I also mentioned earlier that it is the wound of rejection that fuels the most hatred in a person. Why is that? It is because the lack of self-love hurts too much. And the source of this suffering is that what they believe about themselves is the opposite of what they truly are.

**We can see then that hatred is not an indication of meanness, but rather an immense lack of self-love which is reflected back to us by others.**

This is why each time I meet someone who has, or has had, cancer, I know immediately that it is someone who has experienced great disappointment in love. It is the kind of person who wishes so deeply to live in love that, when this love is disappointed, the pain becomes intolerable. They hate their parent of the same sex to the same degree that they hate themselves because what they see in this parent is the same as what they believe about themselves. It is impossible for a person who is indifferent to hate anyone or anything. To hate, one needs to be a very sensitive person.

Furthermore, it is those who suffer from these two wounds who are often considered to be "cold." Particularly adept at hiding their great sensitivity, at withdrawing into their deepest self, these people do not know how to manage their sensitivity. They think that by not feeling, they might suffer less, while actually it makes them suffer more.

It is interesting to make the connection between hate and cancer. We should be aware that there is a huge feeling of powerlessness that hides behind hatred. In the description of cancer we can observe that the body has become powerless to stop the harmful cells from multiplying. It is these same cells that have taken the power and feel all-powerful. They reflect the great power that hatred has taken in the life of the suffering person. This person then receives the message that it is high time they reconnected with their inner power and that they should do so by fostering self-love rather than hatred.

At this stage, you may be saying to yourself, *Is Madame Bourbeau telling us that everyone who hates will end up with cancer?* The answer is *no*. The cancer only develops when this hatred is hidden, when the person is unwilling or unable to be conscious of it, when they deny it and live their pain all by themselves. The person who can acknowledge that they hate their father to the point of sometimes wanting to kill him, will probably not have cancer but could, of course, face another type of illness.

The wound of rejection makes you completely deny that you could have hated your parent of the same sex and the wound of injustice contributes, in its way, to preventing you from expressing this hatred. One of the beliefs of the wound of injustice is the conviction that it is not right, that it is not good, to hate your parents, that you should be a grateful and perfect child. This belief is all the stronger if you give a lot of weight to what a parent may have lost and suffered. Actually, your ego cannot know that if you are afraid to admit you have hated your parents, it will be impossible for you to make a truce with them. Otherwise, a truce could be made once you realize they are in your life to help you become conscious of what you do not accept in yourself.

The rigid and the withdrawer constantly seek perfection but in different ways. The rigid is much more into appearances, into *having* and *doing*, while the withdrawer focuses on *being*, as explained above. The rigid believes they are imperfect if they have to face illness and will have a lot of trouble admitting it, even if they are conscious of it. If they decide to take steps to treat their illness, they will try to conceal the fact. They will even boastingly say that they NEVER take medication and that they NEVER see a doctor.

*Withdrawers*, for their part, deny they are ill at all and therefore don't even see the doctor or don't even talk about what they go through because they also entertain fears at the idea of disturbing others with their problems. You can understand then why withdrawers and rigids cannot feel, or act on, numerous signals they have received from their body before receiving a really big one like cancer.

The more consciously you live, the more you will love yourself and the more quickly you will sense even the smallest signals your body is sending you. Remember that your body is your best friend.

When rigids make a mistake, they will say, *I did not act right, I made a mistake and I will have to do better next time.* The difference with withdrawers is that withdrawers want to BE better. If they make a mistake, they will immediately say to themselves, *I am worthless,* and the next time someone else tells them how to act, they will be convinced again that it is not a comment on their behaviour but on who they are.

***Withdrawers* experience every criticism as relating to who they are rather than to what they are doing. They fail to realize that what they are doing has nothing to do with who they are.**

One of the things motivating the *withdrawer* to develop nervous energy is that it gives him or her a tremendous capacity for work. In their view, the more they *do*, the more they *exist*. It is especially when they are very busy that their existence is real to them. When their wound of rejection is greater, they show nervousness in their gestures and in the way they work. Sometimes they seem to be running in every direction at once.

I must add that although I listed the names of the five wounds, one should not be excessively attached to using these labels. We often use the wrong words to express what we experience. In fact, you can feel rejected by someone who did not keep their promise to you and it may have activated your wound of betrayal.

Your wound of rejection could thus be activated by a situation of rejection, injustice, betrayal, humiliation or abandonment. How can we tell the difference? You can tell by your reaction. Suppose that your husband was unable to keep his promise to you. If your reaction is to say to yourself, *I'm not surprised. It's what I expected. I'm so worthless that it's not important to him to keep his commitment to me,* it shows that it is your wound of rejection that has been activated. The reaction of the wound of betrayal would be to get angry, to accuse your husband openly or to decide never to trust him again. All the characteristics of every wound are further explained in my book and in my workshop on the WOUNDS[2].

## Feeling responsible for others

Over the years, I have noticed that numerous cases of cancer have been discovered among people who thought it was their responsibility to look after their brothers and sisters and even their parents. Several such cases have been found to exist among those who were the eldest child in the family.

In fact, it is not just the *withdrawer* who believes they are responsible for the happiness of others. This belief is present with all the wounds. The big difference is the motivation and the intention.

*Withdrawers* are motivated by a lack of love for themselves, a lack of reasons to live, the lack of a place in life in general and the lack of a sense that they truly exist. Their intention is therefore to fill the void in these areas. Unfortunately, even when

2 Book: *Heal your wounds and find your true self,* published by LES EDITIONS ETC. Workshop: *The five wounds of the soul,* offered by the Listen to Your Body school.

people express genuine gratitude to them, they have great difficulty hearing and especially acknowledging it. They never stop telling themselves that no matter what they undertake, or what they are told, they are still worthless.

**It is impossible to feel the love given by another person if we do not love ourselves.**

Withdrawers often feel they are being held prisoner by others – most of the time unconsciously –, but in reality, they are the prisoner of their belief that they must care for others in order to be *someone*, in order to exist. It is a sad thing, moreover, to realize that they are just going around in circles. They do everything for others in order to exist, but in forgetting themselves, they have the sense that they do not exist.

Even if they were told that no one is responsible for the happiness of another and that it is utopian to think that someone could have that power, the *withdrawer* will not hear it or will deny that he or she feels responsible, saying that everything they do is of their own volition, that it is out of love and not lack of love.

To conclude this chapter, I wish to clarify that the *withdrawer* attracts cancer in order to be shown that he or she must learn to deal with the battle they are engaged in against themselves. After their cancer diagnosis is announced to them, their first reaction is usually to deny it and then, when the wound of injustice takes over, they want to fight against the illness. This is a reflection of their battle against their image of themselves. They are trying to shake off the image they have created of a bad and unworthy person, but since it is only an image, and not a reality, the battle is unwinnable: you can't fight something that doesn't exist.

The cancer is conveying the message that it is now urgent for the person to become aware of their true image and courageously admit all of their qualities and faults in a realistic manner. The next step would preferably be to get assistance from people who know them well and can give feedback as to whether the list is realistic because very likely the perception they had of themselves earlier is still too strong. Isn't this a more pleasant way to live than if you are fighting yourself all the time?

Besides, the word "fight" makes me think of two individuals hitting each other. As they strike one another, their energy gets drained but they keep it up all the same, until one of them, exhausted, concedes defeat. If on the other hand one of them is intelligent enough to stop delivering blows and just follow the movements of the other by moving backwards, the first reaction of the other will be to stop striking. Once the battle has ceased, they will have a much better chance of settling their differences. If you want to be right at all costs, remember that it is always your ego that wants to fight, never the heart. The heart is too intelligent to use such means.

In the final chapter, I will offer other suggestions to assist you further on your path to love, on your path to the unconditional acceptance, rather than the non-acceptance, of who you are.

# Chapter Four

## Why?

This chapter will be divided into three parts in order to deal with the three *why* questions most frequently asked by people who have just learned they have cancer: *Why me? Why now? Why in this part of my body?*

To begin with, the shock of the announcement serves to help the person wake up and become conscious of the damage they have been inflicting on themselves through their thoughts, beliefs and emotions. If they are like the majority of people, who often postpone the important things in life until later, as if they were immortal, the shock will hit them all the harder and they will normally experience moments of panic.

### Emotions and feelings

Let's take a few moments now for a clearer explanation of what is going on with the emotions and feelings. It will certainly help you to understand better why the person who is suffering finds it so hard to be aware of their true feelings. And I truly hope this explanation of the emotions and feelings will also make it easier for you to understand the answers to the three *why* questions that I provide in this chapter.

Cancer is present in the physical body, but since our physical body is the reflection of our other bodies, it means it must have started much earlier, unconsciously. Why is it so difficult to prevent? Because most people don't want to experience their feelings too strongly, believing that they will not be able to manage the pain. But by not feeling, they make it impossible to be really conscious.

**True consciousness is only possible when we allow ourselves to feel what is happening on all levels, in all our bodies.**

When I speak of all our bodies, I am referring not only to the emotional and mental bodies (the material dimension), but also to those of a Causal, Buddhic or Christic nature (the spiritual dimension). The ability to feel resides in your spiritual body while the sensations of these feelings are manifested in your emotional body.

All life has the ability to feel and sense. The difference between humans and other life forms (animal, plant and mineral) lies in the type of consciousness they have. We can know what we feel and sense, which is absolutely necessary in order to be in touch with our intuition. In non-human animals, the feeling and sensing is called instinct. It is what enables them to survive and reproduce. It has even been observed that a flower given and received with love will last and stay beautiful much longer.

The language of feeling is extraordinary and emerges almost instantly. But unfortunately, we are too busy listening to our ego and this interferes with our feeling. The material world has taken too much power over a period of millions of years, ever since humans appeared on Earth. Our material dimension is of course what allows us to live on this planet but, in order to live a harmonious life, that dimension needs to be at the service of our spiritual dimension.

To be more precise, the spiritual dimension represents the part of us that knows all our needs, that knows exactly what we need to live in inner peace and love as well as how to accomplish our life plan. This means then that everything you feel and sense is an indication of the direction in which you are headed. When you feel good in the company of a particular person or in a particular situation, you know you are listening to your needs. If you have an unpleasant feeling, you know right away that what's happening is going against your needs. You can see how important it is to be alert to all your feelings and sensations.

As the wound of rejection is the one that makes us suffer the most, it is normal and human that every time this wound is activated, we cut ourselves off from any feeling and deny that we are suffering. What causes the greatest suffering is the emotions. The feeling, as mentioned above, arises very fast, before we even realize it, and is immediately converted into emotion by our mental activity.

**An emotion is a mental activity of accusation stemming from a fear for self and causing inner agitation**

Whether you are aware of it or not, every emotion is experienced following an accusation. Either you are accusing someone else of rejecting you or you are rejecting someone else in reaction to their not living up to your expectations, or else you may be rejecting yourself because you are accusing yourself of being a failure. There is always a fear for oneself behind every emotion, and it is usually subconscious. What our soul really desires is to feel and experience, without getting emotional. You can achieve this by monitoring how you feel and giving yourself permission to feel either good or not good. A feeling, then, can just as easily have a negative as a positive character, without it disturbing you one way or the other. Getting emotional, however, is always harmful to you, because it drives you to act in a way that is contrary to true love.

Let's take the following example: You have just found out that there has been a family party and you were not invited. You experience it as a personal attack and you suffer because of your wound of rejection which has just been activated. Almost immediately, you start to reject yourself, believing it is your fault and that you are so worthless and unimportant in their eyes that it is only natural that others don't want you there. You aren't even able to think that it might just be an oversight on the part of the host. You close yourself off, you don't say anything and you pretend it doesn't bother you. The feeling of rejection has become an emotion because of your reaction influenced by your wound.

The secret to preventing the feeling from becoming an emotion is simply to observe and note how much you felt rejected by the other person. This will moreover help you to become aware of how much you reject yourself. It is neither good nor bad to feel rejected, it is a human feeling. One day you will love yourself enough to no longer feel rejected so easily. This is an excellent way to live an experience of rejection in acceptance and serenity. The pain would after all only be passing, which is the opposite of what happens with an emotion.

The day you accept that everyone without exception experiences ups and downs, highs and lows, happy and unhappy moments, and that all these experiences are there to help you know yourself and not to make you feel guilty, you will be able to start a new life.

**Accepting every situation, even if you do not agree or do not understand why it is manifesting itself now, is a great act of love toward yourself and toward others.**

Cancer, then, is triggered when the emotional body reaches its limit. An incident occurs that becomes the straw that breaks the camel's back. At the same time, it re-awakens all the other occasions when you tried to hide what you were feeling. The result is that you end up telling yourself, *I can't take it anymore, I can't handle any more of this.* You might even reach a point where you feel so powerless that you think it might even be better to die than to continue having this kind of pain. You can't stand it any longer to be incapable of listening to your true needs. Unfortunately, those feelings are often unconscious.

You will say to me, *But how can I always know what it is I want to be?* If you live more consciously, you will be able to know. Say to yourself every single time you feel uncomfortable in a situation or with a person, *I'm having a problem. It's preventing me from being something I want to be. What am I being prevented from being right now?* It will then be possible for you to discover what you want to be and to decide the actions to take that can help you. We will come back to this subject a little later.

Many of us have a lot of difficulty listening to our true needs because of our ego, which dominates us every time a wound is activated. We spend a good deal of our time then not being ourselves and have come to believe that we are our mental, emotional and physical bodies. They have in the end replaced our *I NEED* and our *I AM*.

This is why you experience so many emotions. You are letting your ego decide, you are allowing it to tell you constantly that this is *good* and this is *bad... expected... right... acceptable* – or not. You are like most people who do not realize how much and how often their mind takes the reins.

## Why me?

People who have just learned that they have cancer will often say things like,

— *Why me? I don't smoke, I watch what I eat, I exercise regularly. I don't understand, especially when I look at my sister who does just the opposite and isn't sick at all.*

— *Why me? I've been attending personal growth sessions for years. I've developed self-knowledge and I thought I had really improved my attitude and made a lot of positive changes.*

These people need to realize that they are not their physical body; nor are they their emotional or mental bodies. Looking after your physical body isn't sufficient. On the other hand, those who stay physically fit are giving themselves a much better chance of healing from their cancer, because they will have more strength and energy to help their immune system recover.

**It isn't what you eat or do physically that weakens your immune system. IT'S THE FEARS YOU HAVE FOR YOURSELF.**

Anyone who has studied their own behaviours and attitudes, and modified certain harmful beliefs, must know that that isn't enough. They must go beyond understanding things. They need first to really be aware of their inner feelings and then to forgive and accept themselves as they are.

This acceptance is made all the more difficult by the fact that it goes completely against what your ego is constantly telling you. The ideal approach is to first reconnect with your inner power and to then, from that place, accept yourself. Over my last thirty years of teaching, I came to realize that acceptance and the notion of responsibility are the two elements of *Listen to Your Body* teaching that provoke the most resistance. It represents something that we were never taught when we were young.

*Why this person and not that one, when I know that everyone has fears?* you ask. *Why did my fears trigger cancer while so many people – who may have even more fears than I do – are not affected?* Here is what I have found to be the answer to that question: it is the degree of hatred that you have experienced toward the parent of the same sex and toward yourself that makes all the difference, and especially the degree of denial of that hatred. Remember that in order to hate, you must have a large dose of love in you. But remember also that if you hate, then this love is not expressed, as it lets itself be hugely controlled by your fears and by what your ego is constantly telling you.

## Why now?

The cancer is showing up now because your inner GOD knows the needs of your soul and considers that you have taken about all you can take. It considers that if you do not want to accept yourself and love yourself as you are now, you will have to face dying in order to return in another life, in a similar or different form, and start all over again. Your inner GOD is giving you a CHANCE to become conscious that it is high time for you to move onto your life path, toward the reason why you are on this Earth, in this environment and in this family. It is just using your body to draw your attention toward this message.

You received countless messages throughout your life but you were too afraid to pay attention to them, to feel what they were telling you. So, you chose to deny them, hoping in this way to avoid feeling the pain of not loving yourself. You sincerely believed you were protecting yourself in order to survive. But remember that this type of belief comes from your ego and not your heart.

I would remind you that the first great hurts, caused by the feeling of being rejected by your parent of the same sex, began manifesting themselves as soon as you were conceived. Since then, you have attracted to yourself several situations and people who have re-activated these hurts. It's as if you were always adding an extra drop to your cup. The fuller it got, the greater the hurts and the more they caused you harm. More and more strength was required for you to be able to tune them out and deny them.

And then it happens. An incident occurs in your life – generally between two and twelve months before the cancer appears – which turns out to be the last straw. The medical world tells you the same thing but in different words. It claims, among other things, that the cancerous cells – called mutations – have been there for years, just like the wound of rejection which, likewise, has been present for years.

Therefore, if you have just found out that you have cancer, I suggest that as a first step you verify what events occurred in your life during the preceding year that caused you stress, pain or emotion. Then verify which of these situations were the most difficult for you to go through, made you suffer the most. By asking yourself what this situation is preventing you from BEING in your life, you will discover that for a very long time you have been preventing yourself from being that way, out of fear of not being loved. This is one of the ways you reject yourself which causes you excessive suffering. Your body is just telling you that you have reached the limit of your endurance, that you have come to the end of your rope, and that you cannot suffer this intensely any longer from this expression of rejection toward yourself.

Let's take the example of the boss who is very tough on his employees. They tolerate it, try their best to do their work while at the same time cursing his meanness under their breath. This situation can be compared to the cells that are trying their best to do their work the way they are supposed to, despite the incorrect codes that they are receiving from their host. One day the employees all meet together and decide to rebel and take over. They don't want to listen to their boss anymore and they do as they wish. This is what happens when the cells decide to take over. They have lost control and anarchy reigns. These cells have reached the limits of their endurance. Clearly it is not the latest incident experienced with their boss that has made the employees revolt, it is the accumulation of several years of unpleasant incidents.

When this cancer was announced, it was a big shock for you, even if only subconsciously. For many people, the shock hits them as if the world has suddenly stopped turning or they are plunging through space after falling off a cliff. This is the effect of the enormous fear that THEIR EXISTENCE MAY END. The suffering part of you may have told you it would be better to die. Or you may have thought, *What use is it to go on living like this?* It is also possible that your will to live has lost its meaning because of all the unfulfilled expectations. Ever since you were very young, you have had to force yourself to believe you existed, because the part of you that suffers was convinced you did not have the right to exist, that you were not important enough.

There are some people who feel such a great emptiness inside, that they subconsciously choose to fill the void with a tumor. This is another way of denying one's feelings.

The phenomenon of synchronicity has also been noted with the appearance of cancers. If for example you have experienced a shock at the death of a loved one, and you were 18 at the time, a cancer could appear 18 years later or when your child reaches the age of 18. Here are some examples of people I have known who experienced this kind of phenomenon. One could also refer to this synchronicity as *memorized biological cycles*.

A man whose father died at the age of 41 when he was only 14 years old, was found to have cancer when *his* son turned 14. A psychologist friend pointed out to him at the time the link between his son's age and what had happened to him when he was 14. After his father's death, he had to become the man in the family, as he was the eldest of the four children, and furthermore had to interrupt his studies to go and work. Being very responsible by nature, he went on to become a big company director. He did not take the time to feel the pain experienced at the time of the loss of his father. But he would still have to do the work of accepting this pain and this loss, because he was angry with his father for having left him when he needed him so much. He had never been conscious of this immense resentment he had toward his father until he received the news of his cancer. He also held it against him that he had not been the model father he sought. Fortunately, he was later healed of his cancer.

Dr. Geerd Hamer did a major study on cancer and explains this kind of situation as a conflict drawn out over many years, which creates a great fear of seeing the same thing repeated later. The fear is all the more harmful as the person is generally not even aware of it. Whenever he or she might begin to sense the fear, they quickly repress the feeling, deny it is there, and do not talk about it. Consequently, they go through it alone and it ends up eating away at them from within.

Dr. Hamer noted then that cancer often appeared after the conflict was over and had been resolved. It was as if the person said to themselves, *Whew, what I was afraid of didn't happen after all. Finally, the problem is resolved and I can relax.*

Here is an example of a woman I knew whose situation corresponds to this same process. She had had breast cancer and it seemed to have gone into remission. I agreed to see her after she learned that the cancer had actually spread to the brain. I had occasion to spend quite some time at her bedside while she was in hospital. When I asked her how she felt about the fact that she might die soon and what it was that she was most afraid of, her reply was, *The only thing I am afraid of is the idea of leaving my daughter. What's going to happen to her?* Her only daughter was 22, a year older than she herself had been when her own mother died.

She learned of her cancer shortly after her daughter's twenty-second birthday. It was as if, ever since her daughter was born, she harboured the fear that her daughter would experience the same pain she had endured because she had never accepted her mother's death. This woman confided to me during my hospital visit that she had never been able to accept it because they were so close but at the same time often had conflict. *Well then,* I said to her, *If you were to die of this cancer, would that mean that you do not love your daughter?* She looked straight ahead of her and did not answer right away. I went on, *The same thing happened with your mother. When she died, it was her soul that made the choice and it certainly was not because she did not love you or rejected you.*

At these words, her face lit up and a big smile appeared, as if she saw something marvellous on the wall opposite her. I knew that she had just felt something of great significance taking place in her. There was so much love in her eyes that I knew she no longer hated her mother for having left her and that she was giving herself permission to leave her daughter. She died a few months later at home, as she was told that this type of brain cancer could not be cured or operated on.

I want to point out again that this whole process happens unconsciously at the time. It is the cancer that finally helps the suffering person to become conscious of it. It is as if their system, constantly under stress and control in order to avoid feeling fear and pain, is finally able to relax enough to give up control thanks to a conflict being resolved. But in doing so, the system goes from one extreme to the other.

Dr. Hamer also recounted the following story. A retired man had lived in the same apartment several years when the landlord told him he would have to vacate in three months because he had decided to rent it out to his son. This announcement sent the man into a panic because he was used to the neighbourhood, felt safe there and had built a life that he was happy with. With no family or friends to help him, he was convinced he could never make a new life anywhere else. He feared he could not find another apartment. He got more and more stressed out and didn't have anyone to talk to about this.

The week before the anticipated departure, the landlord went to meet with the man again, this time to tell him he didn't need to move after all because his son had in the end changed his mind. *WHEW,* the old man said to himself, totally relieved, *it's finally settled and I can continue to lead the life I love.* Two months later, he had stomach pains that got worse and worse. His doctor told him he had stomach cancer. A neighbour, seeing the man's despair, advised him to go and see Dr. Hamer. He had heard that this doctor had discovered a new approach with regard to cancer.

In this approach, it often happens that a person is cured from cancer the moment they realize it is really their body saying it wants to be healed of all the stress accumulated around a certain problem. However, I have observed that this type of conflict resolution in itself is incomplete. The real conflict is inner, not outer. This lets me understand why the cancer reappears – in the same part of the body or elsewhere. Because the conflict has not been resolved in self-love and self-acceptance, but rather by another person, it is finally just an illusion of conflict resolution.

**We must not wait for help from outside to resolve our conflicts. We must rather fulfill our expectations and needs ourselves.**

To come back to the example of the old man about to be evicted by his landlord, we can be sure that he felt quite rejected. However, it is not this rejection that actually caused the cancer. It is all the experiences of rejection that he had experienced since childhood, now being awakened by this specific situation. The fear he felt during the situation with his landlord was just too much. Real healing is therefore only possible when real forgiveness has taken place. I will cover this topic in greater depth in another chapter.

## Fear and its effects

When I learned that adrenalin contributes to causing inflammation, which in turn stimulates the multiplication of harmful cells, I immediately made the connection between fear and cancer. It constitutes another answer to the question *Why now?*

| Effects of fear on the body | Usefulness |
|---|---|
| Higher **adrenalin level** | Provides the extra energy needed to face danger. |

| | |
|---|---|
| Increased **heart rate** | 1) Speeds up blood circulation, thus increasing the oxygen delivered to the tissues while at the same time removing wastes from them.<br><br>2) The blood is also directed away from the parts of the body where its presence is less vital, toward the large muscles such as those of the thighs and biceps, which helps the body to prepare for action. |
| Intensified **breathing** | The tissues need extra oxygen to be ready to respond. |
| Increased **perspiration** | Makes the skin smoother, makes it easier to elude an enemy's grasp, and cools the body to halt any abnormal elevation in the body's temperature (hyperthermia). |
| Other physiological effects:<br><br>1) Dilated pupils<br><br>2) Decreased salivation<br><br>3) Digestive system slowed down<br><br>4) Muscle contraction | 1) Allows more light to enter.<br><br>2-3) Energy conserved for facing potential danger.<br><br>4) Prepare the body for fight or flight, depending on the situation to be faced. |

When a particular danger is perceived or anticipated, the brain sends a message to a part of our nervous system called the *autonomic nervous system*. This system is subdivided into two branches: the *sympathetic nervous system* and the *parasympathetic nervous system*. These two components of the autonomic nervous system are directly involved in controlling the body's energy level and in preparing it for action. To simplify, we could say that the sympathetic nervous system is the one relating to the fight-or-flight response. It frees up energy to enable the body to react. The parasympathetic nervous system is, on the other hand, the one that helps return the body to its normal state.

The chart above illustrates, among other things, the processes that our sympathetic nervous system throws into gear as soon as danger presents itself. It all happens well before our consciousness has a chance to become aware of what's going on, enabling us to either flee or attack. It makes you realize and truly appreciate how intelligently the human species and other animal species have been created. And to think that this automatic phenomenon has been in operation from time immemorial.

This is what people who experience a visceral fear go through for a major part of their lives. The fear I described in the above examples is not a real fear in that there is no imminent danger present. Unreal fear is completely imaginary but the body cannot distinguish between a real and an unreal fear and therefore activates the whole system to prepare to face the anticipated danger.

You understand now why people who live in fear a lot often seem tired. They are actually demanding far too much effort from their system. When someone spends more time in a state of anxiety than in a state of serenity, they produce a lot of adrenalin and moreover wear down their immune system. Scientific research has shown that the immune system is much stronger in a person who is serene and peaceful. Eastern wisdom has known this for a very long time. That is why Eastern medicine is founded on the search for inner peace and balance.

At the same time, I marvel constantly at how strong the body is. Before the cancer or other serious illness shows up, the body has coped for numerous years. It has coped the whole time up until the cells find it impossible to carry out their role properly any longer and lose control.

We can conclude from this that if the cancer shows up earlier in someone's life, it is because the person had stronger fears and was demanding more work from all their systems, causing them to finally weaken. It is moreover possible that these same fears have been experienced over more than one lifetime. In fact, as soon as a system is set in motion, it directly affects the rest of the body. The body is so intelligent that it knows the person's limits and gives the parasympathetic nervous system instructions to take over. With regard to the fears, when the parasympathetic nervous system, whose job it is to bring the body back to its normal state, becomes too worn out, too tired, the person remains in their state of stress and anxiety longer than normal.

We can say then that the behaviour of the person who is more and more afraid, not fully aware of what is going on inside them, and going beyond their limits, is exactly like the behaviour of the harmful cells that keep on reproducing outside their territory and exceeding their limits.

## Why this part of the body?

The place in the body that is affected represents the area of your life that is involved. The physical description of an illness tells us about the life situation the sick person is experiencing.

In my book, *Your body's telling you: Love Yourself!* you will find six hundred different kinds of sickness listed with a detailed explanation of the link between each part of the body and the area of life affected.

When your body speaks to you through the medium of cancer – or any other physical discomfort or sickness –, it is doing so in order to help you become conscious of subscribing to a way of thinking that is not beneficial to you, a way of thinking that prevents you from loving yourself and accepting yourself as you are. Although unconscious, this way of thinking is harming your entire being to the same degree that it is affecting your physical body. When the sickness appears, it is your inner GOD telling you it is high time to change this way of thinking or this unbeneficial belief. It is above all telling you that you have reached your physical, emotional and mental limits.

Your body is playing the role of the little red light that lights up in your car to warn you that there is a problem somewhere. It isn't the little red light that you need to get rid of. You need, rather, to find out what is causing the problem. Otherwise, you'll have a much more serious problem on your hands. And that sounds like most of us: instead of searching for the cause, we just want at all costs to *get rid of* our discomforts and illnesses.

**This light simply wants to draw your attention to something that you are not conscious of.**

Actually, every physical problem helps you discover three important things about yourself:

— An unconscious **need** your soul has;

- A way of thinking (a **belief**) that prevents you from manifesting this need, as well as the **fear for yourself** that has triggered this belief and reinforces it;
- The urgency of **accepting this fear** in order to begin the healing process.

It is important to remember that interpreting an illness is very personal and cannot be determined in advance for everyone. For example, breast cancer does not have the same meaning for each person who struggles with this illness. On the other hand, the area of life represented by each part of the body is generally the same for everybody. We have only to ask ourselves what that particular part of the body is used for in order to see what area of life is involved. For example, a stomach problem is related to someone we cannot digest.

The third message (to accept this fear) is incontrovertibly the most important one. For a long time, I focused expecially on the metaphysical message that explained the psychological cause of the illness. During the last fifteen years, however, I came to understand that the metaphysical aspect was not sufficient. I then oriented myself more towards the spiritual aspect, which means that every discomfort or illness has as its key message **to love ourselves as we are**. By doing so, you become conscious of the spiritual being that you are with your great inner power. It is this lack of love that is the primary cause of all the problems each of us experiences. I would insist therefore on the importance of accepting your fear. It's what proves that you love yourself, that you accept yourself, with your weaknesses.

In summary, once you discover the beliefs that have controlled you and prevented you from manifesting your needs, it then becomes possible to accept yourself, that is, to give yourself the right to have believed in those ideas due to your great fear of suffering or the fear of awakening one of your wounds. And this will in the end be the turning point of your illness.

Many people have difficulty getting through this stage of acceptance because the ego is too strong. The ego does in fact do everything in its power to ensure that you do not accept yourself, because it knows very well that if you stop giving it power, it will starve and become weak. In fact, it has a great fear of disappearing and that is why it resists so strongly. It is moreover convinced it is always right and that if you orient yourself in a different direction and stop listening to it, you will suffer more. I will return to this topic in the last chapter and offer concrete methods for dialoguing with and reassuring your ego.

Here is an excerpt from the book, *Your Body's Telling You: LOVE YOURSELF.* I chose the section on the BREAST because, in most countries, breast cancer is the most common cancer in women.

***EMOTIONAL CAUSES (blocked desires)***

*The breasts have a direct link to the way we mother, whether in relation to our children, our family, our spouse or the world in general. To have a problem with the breast, whether we are a man or a woman, relates to a feeling of insecurity concerning the adequate feeding and protection of those for whose nurturing we are responsible. Nurturing means continuing to treat others as if they were still children dependent on their mother.*

*The breasts also represent the giving of oneself in both our personal and our professional life.*

*For a right-handed woman, the right breast is related to her femininity with a partner. Her left breast is more related to her way of nurturing all those she loves. For a left-handed woman, it is the opposite.*

*If you have a problem with one of your breasts, here are the emotional causes that may apply to you:*

- *You force yourself to come across as maternal in order to be a good parent.*
- *You worry too much about those you love, to the detriment of your own needs.*
- *You unconsciously resent those you love for not having time for you anymore, due to their many commitments.*
- *You are very directing and controlling in your way of mothering.*
- *You mother to the point of being overly cautious.*

*If you are a woman and the problem regarding your breasts is strictly an esthetic one, you are receiving the message that you are too worried about your image. The breasts you have – whether too small or too large – have nothing to do with the amazing person you are. Your body is telling you that you are not your breasts.*

*If it is the breast relating to your femininity, remember that it is only the wound of rejection that is making you fear you are not feminine enough for the man you love.*

### MENTAL CAUSES (fears and beliefs)

*When experiencing a problem related to your way of being a mother or nurturing, you receive a message to the effect that a process of forgiveness needs to be undertaken with your own mother or the person who played that role when you were young. If your way of nurturing is causing you a problem, it is easy to conclude from this that your mother's way of nurturing certainly caused you a problem and was not accepted.*

*Instead of forcing yourself or complaining about what you are going through, it is time to realize that you are not here to protect or nourish all those whom you love. If they ask you for help and you are in a position to give it without going beyond your own limits, that is, while respecting your own needs, do not hesitate to nurture, but do it with love, joy and pleasure. If you cannot or do not want to help, admit this, and give yourself the right to not be able to do it for now.*

*The limits you currently have will not necessarily be the ones you will have all your life. Your sense of duty is excessive and you are asking too much of yourself. You need to learn to let go of those you love. Infants are weaned from the brest not because they have become independent but because, although they still need motherly love, they no longer need the same kind of continual nurturing.*

*If you reject yourself and believe that the slightest couple problem is an indication that you are not very feminine and not beautiful enough for him, it is time you got some clarity on the matter of your femininity through an honest conversation with your partner. You will find out that he does not see things the same way you do.*

### NEED AND SPIRITUAL MESSAGE

*Your great need is to LOVE yourself, to accept the fears you have at this moment. Take the time to find out what you are AFRAID OF FOR YOURSELF in the present situation. Your inner God is inviting you to welcome this fear which is pushing you to act this way, by reminding you that everything is temporary. It is telling you to welcome your present limits and to better recognize your own worth. It is only after accepting yourself in your fears and your limits that you will be able to direct yourself toward what you really want. Remember that it is your ego that is afraid for you, and is convinced it is protecting you. If you feel capable of assuming the consequences of living in accordance with the needs of your being, reassure your ego by telling it that you feel able to assume all possible consequences.*

As you no doubt observed in the metaphysical description of problems related to the breasts, I included several possibilites. It is for you to check and retain what could apply to you.

I want to clarify that if the person with breast cancer is a man, he needs, in addition, to make the connection with the rejection he experienced from his father, his father's way of nurturing. A man's father may have been a very nurturing man, and the man may become a nurturing father himself, but he may have hated his father in that role because he wished his mother had been the more nurturing one. There could of course also be the opposite scenario, where the son decides to become the exact opposite of his father, having always wished his father had been more nurturing toward him.

The best method by far, for discovering as precisely as possible what three messages a particular illness is giving you, is to ask yourself the following questions:

- To discover your need as well as your desires: *What is this cancer preventing me from having and doing (desires) and especially from BEING (your soul's need)?*

- To discover the belief(s) as well as the fear FOR YOURSELF: *If I finally had the courage to direct myself toward what I really want, what could happen to me that would be so terrible? What am I really afraid of for myself? If the object of my fear was realized, what would I be most afraid of? Of being judged as BEING what? Or perhaps of judging myself as BEING what?*

- All you need to do after that is accept this fear for the time being, even if it is preventing you from going toward what you want. By authorizing yourself to be what you are in the present moment, without judging or criticizing yourself, you will be able to gradually reach your goals faster and more easily. You will understand better, when you read the final chapter, how accepting a negative aspect of yourself leads you toward what you want.

It is very possible that your initial reaction to the second message would be a fear for someone dear to you. Let me remind you that in reality, it represents a fear you have for yourself. When this is the case, you need to ask yourself another question: *If what I am afraid of for the other person were to manifest itself, what would I be afraid of for myself?*

To quickly gain a deeper understanding of W*hy this part of the body*, just ask yourself, *What role does that part of my body play in my life*? You may also refer to my book I mentioned earlier, which gives a metaphysical explanation accompanied by a spiritual solution for the great majority of known illnesses.

In the next chapter, you will find more specific explanations of *how cancer begins*, based on real-life experiences.

# Chapter Five

## Learning from real-life experiences

I can honestly say that, over the last thirty-plus years, I have met thousands of people with cancer through the *Listen to Your Body* network, in addition to the numerous cases encountered in my personal life. I have never given a workshop without there being at least one person suffering from cancer at the time or who had suffered from it in the past. What still surprises me is that each of these people seemed to be unaware of the link between their wound of rejection and their cancer, until now.

I personally interviewed several people, including individuals who had taken a number of *Listen to Your Body* workshops and others who hadn't taken any. Those who were willing to answer my questions were deeply moved when they saw the connection with their wound of rejection. All of them consented to let me use part of their story in this book. The cases I selected are presented below.

Please note that all the names used in these examples are fictitious.

### Julie and thyroid cancer

Julie is the eldest in a family of three children who had a very authoritarian mother. The day her mother told her that her father was going to die and that as the eldest she would have to be a support to her and not say anything to her younger sister and brother, Julie decided to obey. She knew that she didn't have to look after them, but found herself all the same incapable of saying this to her mother. At the time, she didn't realize that it was her great fear of being rejected by her mother that made her submissive like this. Although only sixteen years of age, she was required to cooperate and look after the other children. Otherwise her mother would scold her. She was aware that her mother's behaviour was unfair but still decided to keep everything to herself.

Julie was not entitled to express her opinion. When she tried to say something, her mother would order her to be quiet and to go to her room. She didn't dare ask for anything since her mother never came back on a *no*. Rather than having to accept a negative answer, Julie decided very early on to stop asking her mother for anything. She resented her mother a lot for being authoritarian and demanding. She also hated herself for allowing herself to be treated that way by her mother and for continuing to believe that she was not entitled to exist for her own sake, just as she had always believed that she was unimportant. In fact, in the end, Julie believed that she simply wasn't interesting enough, and neither was anything she might have to say.

As an adult, she repeated the same scenario, until the moment she learned she had cancer. When Julie became a nurse, she had a lot of problems relating to one of her colleagues at work. A few months before her cancer appeared, she received an inheritance from her grandmother who had just died. She wanted to stop working so she could focus on looking after her three children.

With news of the inheritance, her husband told her that he too wanted to quit his job. He had always dreamed of starting his own business and the extra sum of money would make it possible. As she had serious communication difficulties and was still unable to give herself permission to listen to her own needs, Julie continued to work, aquiescing to her husband's request, since it was what he preferred. In this example, it is easy to observe Julie's fear of disturbing others when it comes to talking about her own needs, but as well, her belief that in the end, she doesn't really count.

Julie finally quit her job at the age of 40, when she learned she had thyroid cancer. The thyroid gland is related to the throat chakra (a major energy centre) and represents the energy we need to state our wishes or express our will. It represents our ability to take the action required to manifest our needs, and create our life in accordance with our true needs. In short, it is the energy with which we express our creativity.

Later, Julie will admit that, as her father had died of cancer at 40, she had often feared she would get the same illness at the same age. On the one hand, she told herself that she would overcome this illness. On the other, even though it prompted her to stop working, the cancer was preventing her from being herself, from being independent, from being free to decide anything at all, since she had to undergo surgery and several treatments, including radiation and chemotherapy.

To be more precise, Julie received the message to pay attention to the needs of her soul, but also to be herself, to act independently and make her own decisions by taking her rightful place and expressing her needs.

To move through these stages, she had to show compassion toward herself for not having been able to satisfy this need during a good part of her life because she was too afraid of her authoritarian mother and, also, for always being afraid she would not be loved if she decided to put her needs ahead of someone else's. Julie wanted so much to not be like her mother that she went to the opposite extreme and did not express her needs clearly.

Julie had reached the limit of her suffering when she wanted to stop working, but she was unable to express this to her husband. From that point on, everything inside her started to break down and her body showed her it was time to take a break, time for her to finally realize that she was asking too much of herself and that her limits had been greatly exceeded.

Today at the age of 59, Julie is very happy to have done personal growth work and to be able to love herself more by being more attentive to her needs. She knows now that she no longer needs to deny these needs to please others in order to feel loved.

### Nicole and endometrial cancer

The endometrium is the internal lining of the uterus. Its main role is to receive the fertilized egg around the seventh day after fertilization. If there is no fertilization, it is the endometrium which then induces menstruation. As the uterus is the fetus' first home, it is also sometimes referred to as the nest. Uterine cancer is therefore linked to fear, to a feeling of being powerless to properly look after the nest for which we feel responsible. This cancer often shows up in grandmothers who would like everything to go the way they would wish for their grandchildren. It's as if it was their own nest.

In Nicole's case, the child she was concerned about was really an association she had been looking after for almost twenty years. She always considered this association to be her baby. She felt she was a mother to all the members and focused only on their wellbeing. Things went very well until one day a new person joined the board of directors and wanted to change everything. Things gradually began to deteriorate as numerous activities that the members were particularly fond of were cancelled. The turning point came, no doubt, when a final monthly event, which these same members had organized themselves and were looking forward to, was cancelled. The administration decided to keep only the tea dances which interested only those who didn't participate in the other activities. This took place a few months before Nicole's cancer appeared.

Nicole resented this person who was doing everything to contradict her suggestions. As for the other members of the board, who had less at stake, they didn't dare interfere or decide otherwise. Nicole felt she was seeing her baby die, slowly but surely.

In a general sense, what Nicole was going through made her re-live what she had experienced with her mother when she was young. Her mother had been very severe and unbending, and sometimes even violent. Being second in a family of five children, Nicole shared her room with a sister who was three years younger. This sister, in her own way, also caused Nicole many experiences of injustice and rejection. For example, she would lie to their mother and Nicole would be left taking the rap for her sister's misdemeanours. Although perpetually in conflict with her mother and her sister, Nicole kept everything inside and lived her pain in isolation in the hope of keeping peace in the family.

Consequently she experienced the same feeling of injustice in this situation with her association. Since she believed she was responsible for the "nest," she was very much afraid she would be accused of incompetency, of not having carried out her responsibilities properly. She felt the new administration had punished her unfairly, just as her mother used to do. Her intention had been to create a warm and welcoming space for the members. When she felt that she was unable to change what was going on due to a lack of assertiveness on her part, she experienced guilt and self-rejection.

This was another example of someone who had reached their limits, needed to take their rightful place, and decided to do so after their cancer.

Today at the age of 55, and having undergone surgery two years ago, Nicole feels she is cured. She knows now that reconciliation with her mother and sister, as well as forgiving herself, are stages that will be absolutely essential to definitively reverse the consequences of this illness.

By forgiving the parent of the same sex, we also unconsciously forgive all other persons through whose behaviour we experienced the same kind of pain.

## John and prostate cancer

John comes from a family of modest means. A hard worker, he founded a large company that supplies construction materials to contractors. He is especially proud of having done better than his father, who was never very enterprising.

The construction field was very much affected by the economic downturn of the late 90s and several contractors who owed John large sums of money had to declare bankruptcy. One day his bank advised him that he was no longer eligible for the supplementary line of credit. As he faced serious financial difficulties, he had no option but to close down operations and let the financial institution take over his company.

Shortly afterwards, at 78 years of age, he was diagnosed with prostate cancer. The prostate gland represents fatherhood just as the uterus is associated with motherhood. The prostate produces the sperm and, after the ovum has been fertilized by the sperm, the uterus welcomes the fertilized egg and the procreation process in the woman has begun. Furthermore, the word *prostate* derives from a Greek word meaning *to stand in front in order to protect or to shield.*

When a man is placed in a situation where he feels he no longer has the same capability as before to protect his children – especially his son – and if he rejects himself for this, all the elements are present for prostate cancer to appear.

In John's case, during the same period when he found himself in a precarious situation, he experienced great disappointment in his two sons who, in his opinion, were not getting ahead in life, the way he did at their age. When we met to talk about the causes of his prostate cancer, it was with difficulty that John admitted his powerlessness regarding his sons and the future of his company. He experienced strong self-rejection and therefore did his utmost to distance himself from any feelings he might have had about what was going on around him at the time. As a man who had always shown great strength and determination, he went through all this with an acute sense of failure.

To the outside world, though, he claimed he was well satisfied with the turn of events and said that this situation had finally pushed him to take a well-deserved retirement and that he would have no problem living comfortably and happily despite the financial loss he had suffered. Actually, John just wanted desperately for his friends and family not to guess what he really felt. It is another classic example of denial, which so many people choose when confronted by their wound of rejection. I was faced with the obvious truth that as he could not really feel what he was experiencing, John was not in a position to truly forgive himself.

However, I wanted to know if he resented his father for accepting his routine life as a day labourer, not a particularly successful life in his son's eyes. He assured me that in fact he had always loved his father very much and had never judged him. I should add here that John also had a large wound of injustice and that he felt it would have been very unfair of him if he had dared to judge his father. The prostate problem itself diminished, but John died a year later from an aggressive form of bone marrow cancer. All bone problems are linked to a lack of self-esteem and this lack is also associated with the wound of rejection.

In summary, prostate cancer can be occasioned when a son does not live up to the expectations of the father and the father rejects himself for this, believing he was not strong enough to help and protect his son. This cancer can also result if a man lacks or is afraid he will lack money, when he believes that this same money symbolizes his power, symbolizes his image as a good father who sets an example for his children. This explains why so many men end up with prostate cancer shortly after they have decided to take their retirement. When the father feels powerless and useless, he fears greatly that it will undermine his image as a good father. It leads him to reject himself and likewise to be very much afraid to be rejected by his family.

In the example of John, we see an extremely sensitive man who was unable to feel his pain. It was simply beyond his limits to admit that he had felt resentment against his father, that he had rejected him, that he had not wanted to be like him. He said he loved his father very much but it is easy to see from John's lifestyle that he acted in a way that was the exact opposite of his father, which is a sign of rejection.

## Anna and colon cancer

Anna was a middle child with an older and a younger brother. She was taught to be a good little girl and to do as she was told. From a very early age, she felt that her authoritarian mother demanded more from her than from her brothers. And, although she always received good grades at school, her mother never complimented her. Even as a young child, she thought her mother was severe and mean. She was constantly being told she was too young to know what she had to do and should just listen to her mother. Anna therefore felt rejected very early in life and adopted the behaviour of the little girl who rejects herself and obeys in order to be loved.

Until the age of fifteen Anna and her family lived in Africa, but political problems finally prompted her mother to return to France while her father, for his part, decided to remain there. It was a heart-wrenching experience for Anna but her mother did not show the least bit of compassion for her suffering, reminding her instead that it was her duty to obey and follow her mother. It was especially after this that Anna's relationship with her mother began to cool.

Anna and her husband own a flourishing business that has been in operation for several years and today employs 60 people. In 2006, when Anna was 44, one of their employees charged them with workplace harassment. Having absolutely no idea what had prompted this complaint, it was a great shock for Anna. One of the things she asked herself was, *Why me? I have always been kind to my staff. My husband and I have always done everything in our power to make sure our employees were happy to work with us.*

Anna began losing sleep and became more and more depressed. She became obsessed by the whole affair which dragged on for two long years before the courts. Throughout that time, her husband reminded her constantly that they shouldn't talk about the lawsuit to anyone, not even to their family. This made her feel more and more alone in the face of this nightmare. Finally in 2008 they were both convicted by the court, only to be declared not guilty later after they appealed the ruling.

Morally and physically worn down, Anna no longer enjoyed going to work. Moreover, as she was always on guard, she felt like she was in a prison. If she needed to speak to an employee, she made sure there was always a witness, out of fear that the same thing might happen again.

A few months before her cancer appeared in 2010, she and her mother had had a conversation together during which her mother noted that she had been seemed sad in the last while. Anna however denied this and tried to make her mother believe that everything was going just fine at work, with her husband and with her two boys. Her mother sensed that there was something serious going on and so she insisted. Anna then ended up admitting to her all that she had gone through since 2006.

When her mother learned they had been found guilty by the court, she did not react at all the way Anna had hoped. She actually expected her mother to understand her and support her in her anguish over this. Instead her mother was more interested in understanding the employee's motives for taking them to court. This reaction was the last straw for Anna. In fact she hated herself a lot for continuing to expect better from a mother who treated her so coldly and so often made her feel rejected.

When she learned of her cancer, it represented of course another major blow for her. The doctor gave her this news by phone on a Friday evening and added that she should be at the hospital the following Monday because her case was very urgent. It was a stage three cancer. She felt completely deflated, just like when she found out she would have to move back to France without her father; just like when she found out one of their employees was taking them to court; just like when she and her husband were convicted; just like when she heard her mother's reaction to learning of all the problems her daughter had faced in the last three years.

It is not difficult to see the connection between all these incidents. But why did Anna attract cancer in precisely that place in her body, in the colon? Here is an excerpt from the book, *Your Body's Telling You: Love Yourself*, explaining the metaphysical aspect of the *colon* and the *large intestine*:

*A problem in the large intestine develops when you have difficulty letting go of your old ideas and beliefs that no longer serve you (constipation) or you reject ideas too quickly that could be beneficial to you (diarrhea). You are so afraid of things that annoy you and are beyond your control, that you simply cannot stomach them. You are probably the kind of person to say someone is "a pain in the ass" before seeing the positive side of the person or situation that evokes your fear of scarcity or that you fear will waste your time.*

*Your intestinal problem is an important message. It is saying you must re-learn to nourish yourself with good thoughts, not feed yourself fears and demeaning thoughts. Also, you no longer need to believe in scarcity in your material world. You must above all work on your faith; have faith in a divine presence in you and in the Universe which is there to look after all life on this planet, including you. You must let go of the old in you to make room for the new.*

The description given above applies to any condition or illness related to the colon. However, when it is cancer we are talking about, in a specific part of the body, it means the message is much more serious and urgent than when there is just a general problem in that area. The cancer has been present from very early on in childhood and, as it has been ignored for so long, the cumulative layers of pain begin to exceed the person's limits.

Anna therefore needs to get in touch with the constant suffering that has made her feel so insecure and afraid of losing someone or something dear to her. To ensure that there will not be a relapse, the next thing she needs to do is to reconcile with her mother and forgive herself for often being what she judged and didn't accept in her mother. She will have to develop self-esteem rather than wanting the absolute approval of others. When she accepts that she has limits and the right to not always be nice and have to obey, she will be on the road to becoming what she wants to be. In the end, she will have the pleasant surprise of discovering the special woman she is, a warm-hearted woman of many talents, even if she isn't always what she would like to be.

## Richard and leukemia

Richard comes from a family with two children. His father was very protective of his older sister while, toward Richard, he acted particularly cold, demanding and directive. Since his father ran the family business that he had inherited from his own father, Richard thought that if he went to work with him, it could help them become closer.

He soon realized, however, that this decision hadn't helped at all, far from it. Just as demanding as before, his father wanted him to learn everything about the business, making him work in each department. Richard didn't necessarily mind the various tasks, but at the slightest little error, his father would berate him publicly, in front of the other employees. Richard thus felt more and more rejected, although he was doing everything to please his father and especially to gain his approval, his efforts went unrewarded. His father always remained dissatisfied. Even when he married at the age of 22, it was to please his father.

Finally having had enough, despairing and feeling powerless to change anything at all in his relationship with his father, he decided after a few years (at the age of 27) to leave everything behind and go and work in Africa. During the process of having all the required vaccinations and bloodwork done, it was discovered that he had leukemia. He learned furthermore that there was no treatment for it and he had no more than 10 years left to live. Since he didn't really feel sick and saw no point in undergoing painful examinations on a regular basis to monitor his illness, as the doctors had advised him to do, Richard decided that if he was about to die anyway, he would make the most of these last years remaining to him.

First, he gave himself permission to divorce. That was a difficult decision for him. It was the first time he was undertaking something for himself, daring to take the risk of truly displeasing his father. He had to countenance the same words he had heard over and over from his father since he was young: *You will be the death of me yet!* As well, Richard began to smoke and drink a lot more and to eat whatever he felt like. He had been so careful as a young man never to indulge even the smallest of his whims – because his father demanded perfection of him in all things –, that he gradually veered to the other extreme in reaction.

During those ten years, Richard never once went for a health checkup. Noting that he was after all still alive at the end of this period, he did however finally go back to his doctor to have a blood test. He learned to his great joy that he no longer had cancer. Not actually feeling very fit due to all the excesses he had allowed himself over those last years, he decided to lead a more balanced life. He started working on personal growth and living a healthier lifestyle.

Since Richard had been prevented from going to Africa because his immune system was too weak and he could not have the vaccinations, he decided to continue working with his father. Despite the news of the cancer and the healing, nothing in his father's attitude had changed.

The father suffered from a wound of rejection just like his son. He simply wanted to deny the fact that his son only had 10 years to live. In fact, the more Richard tried to prove to his father that he was neither stupid nor useless, the more he did things that made his father consider him incompetent. His decisions were poorly timed and he often showed poor judgment, inevitably entailing serious consequences for the company.

The "biggest bloody mistake" he'd ever made, he said, was the time he let himself be conned by a crook with whom he had invested large sums of money. It put him in debt for twenty long years. This bad decision occasioned still more rejection from his father, who showed his disappointment in no uncertain terms. He continually told his son that he definitely had potential but that he did not know how to use it. He often compared him with his sister, saying, *Look at your sister. You have more talent than she does and you're not amounting to anything*. All Richard was trying to accomplish here was to show his father that he could succeed on his own. So he kept on hearing how incompetent he was. This is how it goes with all of us when we are influenced by our wound of rejection.

**The more we are afraid of being rejected, the more we behave in a way that invites rejection. It becomes a vicious circle.**

Coming to the end of his career and suffering from health problems, Richard's father resigned himself to taking his retirement five years later. Richard knew that his father would let him take over the reins of the company, albeit reluctantly, and that he still did not have confidence in him or in his abilities. And yet, Richard handled the business very well after that. Did that change what his father had always thought of him? Absolutely not! He even reproached Richard for having become a wheeler-dealer.

Feeling his deeper values to be more and more at odds with the business world, Richard decided after twelve years to step down from his duties. He sold the company to some of its executives and another family member.

He finally understood that what had helped cure his cancer was the decision to want to live and to recognize his own value, instead of waiting for recognition from his father. Richard is now over 60 and thanks to all the inner work of reconciliation and forgiveness that he has done with himself and with his father, he has doubly assured himself that there will be no relapse.

### Denise and cancer in the right breast

Denise was another person who felt very much rejected throughout her entire childhood. Yet, she was the eldest of three children and her parents awaited her arrival with eager anticipation. On the other hand, her mother always controlled everything and Denise never felt free to do what she wished or to say what she thought.

Very early on, Denise learned she should always make her mother happy if she wanted to feel loved. She moreover always believed she was the least loved of the children – her brother and sister being loved more. This is why she went to such great lengths to earn her mother's love. The mother, who rejected herself also, never wanted to be called *mom* and asked her three children to call her *Kitty.*

Once when she was about eight years old, Denise dared to call her mother *mom*. Clearly angered by this, her mother looked at her with an icy stare. Even forty years later, Denise can still feel the shiver it sent through her. From her mother's reaction, Denise knew never to use the word *mom* again. It is easy to see that her mother was a woman who never wanted to accept her maternal role.

This sort of case is commonly found among women who refuse to be like their own mother because they are afraid of losing their femininity and thus losing their husband's interest as they take on the role of mother. It is unfortunate that many women believe they cannot play both roles, that of spouse and that of mother at the same time, that they need to be one or the other, which is clearly false. The jealousy Denise could feel coming from her mother whenever her father granted her privileges is another indication of her mother's fear of losing her husband.

The same scenario repeated itself in Denise's life. She in effect never wanted to imitate her mother's behaviour and did her utmost to be a better mother. She was very maternal with her children, believing that in this way she was being different from her own mother. However, she constantly experienced the conflict created by her decision to be different from her mother and by the belief that if she wasn't nurturing enough toward her husband, she might lose him.

Since she began living more consciously after she learned she had cancer, Denise realized that she too was sometimes jealous of her daughter, like her mother was.

She and her husband were a couple who loved each other very much, but her husband had been struggling with an addiction problem for several years. Denise thought it best to join him in this dependency because she felt he was slipping away from her when he was under the influence of drugs. This problem evolved into a conflict affecting their life as a couple, as she was begging him to stop time after time so that she herself could stop. She felt incapable of stopping of her own accord and hated herself for this weakness. The fear of losing her husband was obviously stronger than her desire to live up to the image of a good mother.

A few months before the cancer appeared in her right breast, a trigger event took place. When, after begging him once more to stop, her husband told her he had no intention of quitting, she felt a deep anger toward him. He added that he felt no guilt over this dependency and that it suited him well for the time being. She then shot back at him with, *So, will I have to be half-dead before you realize the harm your habit is doing me?*

Unconsciously, she had just said that it was only if she almost died or even did die, that her husband might finally recognize the danger of his drug habit and have an incentive to stop.

It was her wound of injustice that led Denise to accuse herself of being absolutely worthless in this situation. She lived with guilt and shame for many years and even quit her job as a therapist because she considered herself unworthy of acting in that capacity given the kind of weakness she had. This self-rejection awakened the self-rejection she had experienced with her mother when her mother insisted she become a nurse while Denise wanted to be a doctor. She felt rejected at the time, convinced that her mother didn't consider her good enough to have a career as a doctor; she felt that her mother didn't want her to be better than her. This made her feel like a total failure.

Denise knew that her mother was very close with her husband and wanted at all costs to be the ideal woman to him while still having a family. Unfortunately she chose to deny herself the experience of being maternal, in order to continue assuming her spousal role as perfectly as possible. In the end she became a directing and controlling mother instead of a nurturing one. I am speaking here of Denise's perception for I am certain that her mother was convinced she was a good mother.

Not wanting to be like her mother, Denise did everything possible to be very nurturing, which at the same time awakened her fear of losing her husband. Using drugs with him was an opportunity to be present, close and seductive.

Denise was among those who, after the initial shock of the cancer diagnosis, wondered, *Why me? I watch my health and I've been a vegetarian since I was young. I've even done a lot of inner work. I just don't understand.*

Actually, she was simply receiving the message that she needs to accept herself in the reality of being a mother like her mother, even if at times her behaviour is different, and to make her peace with that truth. Her body was showing her that she had reached her limit, that she would find true happiness in her life when she accepts herself as she is.

If you see yourself as a person who does not want to be like your parent of the same sex, it is an indication you accept neither that parent nor yourself and this is a manifestation of rejection. **All the time that you take to not be like this parent leads you to be another person who, unfortunately, does not meet the needs of your being.** The parent of the same sex as you, who was chosen by you before your birth, is the most important person in your incarnation. He or she is in your life to help you become conscious of what you do or do not accept in yourself.

**You must remember above all that when you feel rejected by your parent of the same sex, you are rejecting this parent just as much and they feel this rejection just as much as you do, even if this happens unconsciously in each of you.**

## Joan and cancer in the left breast

Joan is the fifth of twelve children and comes from a dysfunctional family that saw violence and love play out in turn. It was the kind of home where children can no longer tell what is up and what is down. At a very young age already, Joan's self-effacing nature was apparent. She was docile and helpful and did her best in order to be loved. She didn't dare cry because she was afraid her mother would hit her to make her stop. That's what her mother had done other times.

At the age of eight, she witnessed a particularly violent scene one day. She saw her father hold a knife to her mother's throat, threatening to kill her if she didn't admit she had cheated on him. She was so afraid her mother would die and be gone forever that she vowed then and there to look after her younger brothers and sisters as a way of preventing anything so terrible from ever happening again. Being an alcoholic, her father often went into fits of rage. Joan made this promise because in her child's mind, she believed her parents were fighting because of the children. She didn't understand what her father meant by "cheated." She told herself that if she took very good care of the children and they all behaved well, it would keep this kind of situation from happening in the future.

The family unit was what mattered most to Joan. She protected it constantly because it was only through it that she felt she existed. This meant she often took her mother's place doing the household chores, since her mother was away a lot. In fact, her mother went out to play bingo seven times a week. Joan ended up doing everything – cleaning house, preparing meals, babysitting the youngest ones, etc. She admits today that keeping busy like that was one way for her to be able to know that she really existed. Remember that when the wound of rejection is activated, we truly believe that we do not have the right to exist.

She noticed also that her mother was quite capable of one day behaving in a very nurturing way with all her children and the next day acting as if they were too much for her. As far as Joan was concerned, she always wished she had a mother who could be nurturing all the time. Yet at the same time, she did not like her mother's way of being nurturing.

In her adolescent years, Joan began asking herself, *What am I getting out of struggling like this? She doesn't love me any more for it, and she doesn't give me any recognition either.* She had wanted more than anything for her mother to love her, but then began to detest her. She told herself she would suffer less that way; it would be less painful than to love her so much and see that she didn't even exist for her. From then on, she often wished her mother would die.

What she held against her the most was her attitude to her father. She pampered him continually, forgave him everything, and looked after him despite his alcoholism and his violent outbursts. And she acted the same way with her sons, while her daughers were expected to serve the men in the house. Consequently, she found her mother very unfair. At the same time, she silently resented the fact that her mother did not stand up for herself and command respect. Not wanting to be like her mother, Joan of course had her own reasons for looking after her younger brothers and sisters. She wanted to show her mother that she was better than her.

She married, gave birth to a boy and two girls and kept up her mothering role not only toward her own children but toward her brothers and sisters too, doing everything for them. Even when she felt her efforts were not recognized, she continued to act in this way as it was the only way she knew to feel she really existed and to seek love. This way, she was also keeping her promise to herself to be a good mother. She didn't realize at the time that all this was just as much a reaction against her mother.

When her children were 11, 10 and 6, Joan divorced her husband. She had to take three jobs to make enough to support her children and was therefore often away. When her children were grown, she began a job that required her to be out of the country for periods between one and three months. She felt guilty about having to be away that often and was therefore extremely permissive whenever she was back, even tolerating the irresponsible behaviour of her son who would squander his money and always seemed to be running short. As Joan had still not accepted her mother's behaviour, she was unaware that she hated herself for being the same kind of mother and kept telling herself that she was doing it out of love for her children. She was even proud of being such a good mother.

There were two incidents that had a strong influence on Joan shortly before her cancer appeared. The first took place during one of her trips. She had entrusted her ex-brother-in-law and her son to carry out some renovations to the house while she was away. Upon her return she learned they had significantly exceeded the budget she had set and furthermore that a lot of the work had been sloppily done. This meant that she had to hire other contractors to re-do the unsatisfactory work, which added still more to the cost.

The second incident arose when she discovered that her daughter, who had a partner and two children, had rented the second apartment of their home to her father, Joan's ex-husband. Her daughter had promised her mother she would keep the apartment for her so that she could live there after her house was sold. Joan had been planning for some time to put her home on the market, because the idea of being near her daughter made her very happy, especially as she adored her grandson and would then be able to pick up her "mothering" role once again.

Sometimes when she had just returned from a long trip and was suffering from jet lag, she would still agree to look after her grandsons to make her daughters happy. When she learned her daughter had decided to rent out the apartment to her father, she took it as another low blow, as he had hardly ever paid attention to the children since the divorce. This situation evoked in her the fear that her daughter might prefer her father, reminding her of the injustice she had experienced from her mother.

Joan was 59 when she received the news that she had cancer. Nine months later, she agreed to have her sister and brother come and live with her, claiming it would feel safer to have someone living at the house whenever she was away and that she could look forward to company each time she returned. What she did not dare to admit to herself, though, was that their company was more inconvenient than helpful and that she didn't feel respected. But as a typical *withdrawer* (wound of rejection), she went right ahead in her mothering role and let a lot of things go without comment. She sometimes got angry with her brother and gave him a piece of her mind, but it was wasted effort. He did not change his habits and she continued to accept the situation.

When Joan learned she had cancer, she was naturally beside herself. She felt it was so unfair after how much she had been looking after herself for several years – physically by watching her diet and psychologically by doing personal growth work. She looked for a doctor who would agree to remove only the tumour so that she would not have to go through chemotherapy but they all refused. So she decided she would heal herself. Following the biopsy done on her breast, a wound gradually formed and fluid began to seep out from it.

She tried to understand the message her body was sending her, took good care of herself, ate in a very healthy way according to the new raw and living foods diet she had learned about and drank only the healthiest juices. She followed various cures and fasts, did several weeks of meditation, but in vain. A year later, the wound remained and was even somewhat larger. She had to face the fact that she was stuck in denial.

In the meantime, her brother was still living with her, her sister had left after a few months and her ex-husband still lived in the apartment in her daughter's house. Her son came to see her regularly to complain about his problems and ask for money. As things stood, the situation had hardly improved, but revealed to her, at the same time, that she was going beyond her limits and it was becoming urgent that she feel, at long last, what was happening inside her.

Although little improvement could be noted in either her cancer or her wound, Joan continually demonstrated a lot of energy for her personal affairs, her work and her numerous trips abroad. It seemed like she was getting a boost from the Universe, which in my view, was the reward reaped from all the efforts made over the previous eighteen months despite her illness.

The turning point came when she arrived home one day from one of her long business trips and discovered that her brother had once again abused her hospitality and engaged in illicit activities in her home. Instead of going into denial as she had done in the past, she finally realized, identified and felt how great was her lack of self-respect and understood how that made it impossible for her to command respect from others.

When I asked her to describe that wound that wouldn't heal, what it was like to experience that, here is how she replied: *It is like an intruder. It takes up more and more space. It nibbles away and makes me suffer. It's like something is pulling on me and sometimes it feels like I'm being stabbed. The pain wakes me up at night, it's all-consuming, very disturbing. I feel invaded and powerless. I can't get a good night's sleep or live a normal life; I can't find inner peace and serenity or feel joyful and confident.*

The words she used to describe the wound are exactly the words that describe the situations she had been enduring for a long time and did not want to see. With her wound of rejection, she even denied having felt invaded and powerless in the incidents that took place shortly before she received the news of her cancer. She began to discover what her body was most in need of: to create a life of calm, joy and confidence. To achieve this, she would need to stop having her family and friends invade her privacy. She wasn't achieving it because her ego was convinced that if she behaved that way in order to find serenity and joy, she would be excluded by those she loves.

She remembered feeling excluded and therefore rejected by many people ever since she was a small child. Men and women who didn't want to see her anymore because she mothered them too much. It is easy to see here how much our ego plays tricks on us. Have you ever noticed that the more you bend over backwards to not be a certain way, the more you are that way? In Joan's case, she was mothering in order to be included but the more she was motherly the more she was excluded. What a paradox! This revelation opened the door wide into the realm of consciousness for Joan. She was finally able to feel the pain she had always lived with as she nurtured others in her motherly way.

It is obvious that Joan's main goal has always been to feel loved. She has still not come to realize that she needs above all to love herself, and that love from others would follow quite naturally.

**We cannot receive from others what we do not give ourselves, just as we cannot give to others what we do not possess.**

What is more, she could finally feel what her mother had experienced, since she too let her children and her husband exploit her, and how impossible she found it to stand up for herself. She could finally feel her mother's pain and her own and how each of them rejected themselves to the point of forgetting themselves completely for the sake of their loved ones. They believed that their mothering would make others love them and would give them the right to exist.

As I write these lines, a few weeks after the work we did together, Joan's pain is diminishing little by little. Her brother finally went to live elsewhere and her son has gotten into the good habit of phoning before stopping by at the house. In fact, she agrees to see him as long as it is not to solve his problems. She established her limits with them, just as she did with her ex-husband while accepting the need he expressed to see his children and grandchildren.

Today, she thanks her body and the message that came through her breast cancer, for having helped her undertake a huge labour of love for herself. It is up to her to continue to act out of love for herself and not out of fear of illness, as the latter would be indicative of her fear of not being loved by others.

## The difference between cancer in the left breast and cancer in the right breast

For a right-handed woman, cancer – or any problem – in the right breast is related to her femininity as experienced with her spouse. She refuses to be like her mother, absolutely wants to be a better mother, and remains unaware that she quite simply shares the same fear her mother had: she is afraid this mothering will cost her her femininity, and in the process, her husband too. For a left-handed woman, it is the opposite.

For a right-handed woman, cancer in the left breast is related, rather, to her way of nurturing all those she loves. She does her utmost to not be like her mother, even though she and her mother have many similarities, something each of them denies.

For a left-handed woman, the last two descriptions are reversed.

In both cases, everything the woman does is with the intention of being a much better mother than her mother and, although she is like her mother, she is convinced she really is better.

## Summary of these real-life experiences

You will surely have noted several similarities as you read the descriptions above. In each case,

– The parent of the same sex is described in similar terms: demanding, severe, authoritatian, unjust, categorical, often violent...

- The children are docile, loveable and good, and do everything to make this parent happy, at the same time having the impression that it is never enough.

- They deny their pain and succeed in making themselves believe that their parent of the same sex loves them, until the day when they rebel. If they really felt loved, they wouldn't be bending over backwards to win their love.

- They become an adult prematurely, assuming responsibilities that are not theirs.

- They do not manage to express what they feel. They are convinced they are not entitled to give adults their opinion. They choose therefore to deny what hurts them or what might cause someone else to be hurt.

- Out of fear of being refused, the children have a lot of trouble asking for anything and this represents more rejection.

- They find it very difficult to be able to take their rightful place and often choose to be alone.

The traits listed above are actually the typical behaviour of anyone influenced by their wound of rejection. If you recognize yourself in this description and you tell yourself you did not feel rejected by your parent of the same sex, it is very possible that you used different words to describe your relationship with this parent which excluded the words *reject* and *rejection*. It remains nevertheless true that the pain will have been just as great, even if you used other words to describe it.

**The trait most likely to sow the seed of cancer from a young age is living the pain of feeling unloved in isolation. Children who experience this deny what they are going through and cannot talk about it to anyone because they are unconscious of it themselves.**

I met a woman who stated categorically that she had never experienced rejection by her mother. She added that her mother did all she could for her children. However, this same woman admitted that she had experienced a lot of anger toward her mother and had often rejected her, wanting more than anything not to be like her. In fact she was unable to admit the notion of the mirror which states that *"the way we experience another person is also the way that person experiences us."* So here is another example of denial experienced due to that very painful wound.

It is true that a great many parents who are strict, demanding and unfair commonly tell their children that they treat them this way because they love them. And it is just as true that a child who lacks love will choose to believe that, rather than have to admit that they do not feel loved. The child is not yet wise enough to know that if they do not feel loved, it is simply because they do not love themselves. Their parent is only acting this way toward them to reflect back to them their lack of love for themselves.

It is also possible you are recalling that you were not always docile and obedient as a child and were sometimes given to fits of anger. In that case, it is your wound of injustice that took over. Also, remember that in this book, I am speaking mainly about pain experienced with the parent of the same sex. Whenever you experienced difficult situations that made you resent the parent of the opposite sex, it is the other wounds that were involved.

There is also a strong likelihood that if you are convinced you felt much more rejected by the parent of the opposite sex than by the parent of the same sex, it is another trick your ego wants to play on you. It is trying to make you believe that it is your parent of the opposite sex that you hate more, but I invite you to go deeper. I have witnessed numerous cases where a person like you has ended up admitting that they hated their parent of the same sex more for not having defended them when the other parent hurt them physically or psychologically.

All those fits of anger you had when you were young may have helped you reduce the accumulation and repression of things inside you, which is what causes cancer. We often hear people say that cancer is like a little beast eating away at us from inside. The "little beast" actually represents the bitterness and hatred that we do not want to see and that we keep repressed inside.

People who let it all out by using anger and accusations toward others will for their part attract illnesses other than cancer. The person with cancer experiences a lot more anger toward themselves because they see themselves as the parent of the same sex whom they refuse to accept. They will go very much out of their way to not be like them.

As soon as they become conscious of all that repressed anger and their great pain stemming from rejection, that's when healing can start. But healing cannot really take place until they can forgive themselves and their parent of the same sex. This will be the subject of the next chapter.

# Chapter Six

## Forgiveness: the one and only solution

Those who are familiar with the teaching of *Listen to Your Body* will hardly be surprised at the title of this chapter. It is possible, however, that if you are new to this kind of approach – metaphysical and/or spiritual – you may demonstrate a certain resistance. I want to remind you that this is perfectly normal. I can still remember the resistance I felt when I started to open up to certain things. I got started on this process through studying and practising positive thinking. It's what was being taught in the field I worked in at the time, namely, sales.

I was then ready to want to learn about new things but my ego did not agree with my *I NEED*. For my part, I considered that the idea of being able to manifest everything that we wanted seemed too good to be true. At that point in my life, I still believed in good luck and bad luck. When however I started having very good results thanks to positive thinking and the programs I was following on a regular basis, I finally let go.

A few years later, a friend put me in touch with someone from California who gave a talk that was, to say the least, different and more spiritual. When I heard the speaker say, *I am God and we are all God* right at the start of the talk, I could feel strong resistance rise up in me. I had a lot of difficulty letting go and just *being* with what he was saying, without judging it as good or bad. A little voice in my head said, *Who does that guy think he is, making statements like that? He will have to provide proof if I am to believe him. How can he declare that we, as GOD, are so filled with love that we can forgive regardless of the wrong that was committed?*

The speaker told of the numerous healings he had witnessed when people reconnected with their inner power and with love. It was only through attending more spiritual lectures over the following year that I really began to understand the message this man wanted to convey to us. When I met him later, there was no more resistance on my part. He had in the meantime created a very large centre in Southern California and it is at this school that I earned my bachelor's degree in philosophy.

After so many years and thousands of testimonies from our participants, it is certainly easier for me today to have a more open vision and to be totally convinced of what I advocate.

**I KNOW now that it is true that healing can only take place with the help of forgiveness and self-acceptance.**

Unfortunately, the word *forgiveness* often makes people react a certain way. For some, it has a religious connotation while it reminds others of submission. Several of them say, *If you forgive, it's like saying the other person was right to treat you that way. It's the other person who should be asking for forgiveness! I have nothing to forgive myself for, when it is other people who rejected me and made me suffer. How can Lise Bourbeau say that just the fact of forgiving oneself is enough to heal a disease that medicine hasn't managed to cure after all these years of research?*

Whether in my workshops, my talks or any of my books, I have never promised or stated that a person was going to be able to heal themselves. I can however state that a very large number of people have healed themselves, and that others have not, depending on what they have put into practice in their lives. It is important to make a distinction here: we are talking especially about work done in the sphere of the soul's path to inner peace. Any inner work we undertake is never lost.

All this is to say that you have nothing to lose and EVERYTHING to gain by being willing to reconcile with those whom you have accused of making you suffer and especially by forgiving yourself. If you feel resistance in yourself, welcome it, knowing that it is normal and human to have trouble with any spiritual notion. Remind yourself that it is not your heart that is resisting but your ego. It cannot comprehend this kind of notion. Next, give yourself the time you need to work through all of the following stages.

## Responsibility and acceptance

In order to put the odds on your side, you must first accept the fact that everything you have created in your life comes from within you. It is what we call "the notion of responsibility." *Being responsible* means knowing that you are constantly creating in your life, according to your actions, reactions, interpretations and decisions, regardless of what the situation is. You know that you are being responsible when you are able to accept that whatever you do or are, you do not have to feel guilty, because you will always be the one who must assume the consequences.

In summary, taking responsibility is the antidote to guilt.

**To be responsible is to recognize that every action has an effect and that it is thanks to its consequences that we become conscious of what is or is not intelligent for us.**

To be responsible is to recognize that every action has an effect and that it is thanks to its consequences that we become conscious of what is or is not intelligent for us.

**To accept is to acknowledge, to welcome and to observe a fact, without any judgment, either good or bad.**

As soon as you accept, you become centered. **To become centered means to return to the light.** Consequently, to be uncentered – when you let your ego do the directing – distances you from the light. Remember that the more uncentered you are, the more you will find yourself in a kind of haze that prevents you from seeing situations and people as they are. This absence of light limits you moreover in your ability to recognize the needs of your being.

When you are unable to accept a situation or a person and you want to change them because you cannot accept them, it is as if you were standing in front of a door and you were pounding it with your fists in an effort to open it. You do not see that there is a handle to open it because you have your nose to the door. You perceive the door as a wall standing in your way. The harder you pound, the more harm you do yourself.

Acceptance can be compared to stepping back from something, looking at a situation as it is and realizing that that door has a handle and that all you have to do is turn it and the door will open with ease. Acceptance thus leads you to new horizons so that you are no longer a prisoner of your fears. It prevents you from doing yourself harm and panicking.

To help you follow the various stages of reconciliation and forgiveness, I will use the example of Denise whom I accompanied as she progressed through them.

## Accusations and emotions

Here is a description of the first stage in the achievement of self-forgiveness. Let us go back to the example of Denise. She takes a few moments to wind down and relax. She knows now that the day she got so angry with her husband because he would not quit his addiction (the day she said, *Will I have to be half dead before you see the harm your drug habit is doing to me?*) awakened in her all the anger she had toward herself for not standing up to her mother and being like her mother, who also did whatever it took to hold onto her husband.

She closes her eyes and reviews all the accusations she made against her mother for who she was, all the things she accused her of *being*. She then notes down on paper what came to her during that exercise:

— *I accused my mom (until now) of being controlling, manipulative, unfair, egotistical, spiteful, weak and fragile.*

Next, she reviews how she felt with a mother who acted weak and fragile with her husband while at the same time being unfair with Denise. She notes on her paper:

— *I felt rejected, sad, angry, despairing, misunderstood, not listened to, alone, isolated from the whole family. I felt I had no right to exist as me.*

**One cannot be fully conscious of a situation without feeling what is going on inside. Without feeling, it is just analysis.**

When you do this kind of work and have trouble putting your feelings into words, it is because you didn't fully experience your anger. There is ALWAYS anger in every painful situation a person experiences.

Keeping your eyes closed, take the time to check in what part of your body this anger is located. How intense is it on a scale of 1 to 10, ten being the angriest you could ever be?

*Denise experiences the anger in her throat, reminding her of her inability to express herself or to get her mother to listen. The intensity is 8 on a scale of 1 to 10.*

Next, allow to rise up in you everything that accompanies this anger, giving yourself permission to fully feel what is taking place in you when you suffer. It is only by feeling and fully accepting this anger that you will be able to feel the other emotions that are hiding behind it and especially to feel the fear of rejection. You must take the time needed to discover as many of your accusations and emotions as possible.

Look at the anger in you and accept the idea that it is normal and human to have this kind of anger when you suffer. To be angry does not mean that you're a bad person. On the contrary, it shows that you're a sensitive person and that you're capable of feeling suffering, which is an indispensable stage if it is to be healed. Fill this space – where your anger is the most concentrated – with white light and take a few deep breaths. At this point, you are ready for the next stage.

## Fear for yourself and expectations

Now that Denise is conscious of the accusations she made against her mother and against herself and is conscious of everything she felt and experienced, she can move on to the stage of reviewing all the fears she had for herself in the situation concerning her husband.

An important thing to remember is that in any unpleasant situation, you are always afraid for yourself. Your ego on the other hand makes you believe that you are afraid for others. In Denise's case, she believes she is afraid for her husband, afraid of what may happen to him, especially if his addiction gets even worse.

**The real fear is the one we have for ourselves and not the fear we have for others.**

Denise therefore starts to note down the fears she has for herself at the moment of an angry outburst.

— *I'm afraid that I will die if I continue to keep him company in his addiction. I'm also afraid that if I stop drinking and am no longer capable of watching him harm himself, I will finally decide to leave him. I'm afraid of losing the true love that we have experienced, of destroying the family unit, of facing financial uncertainty and seeing the cherished family life that we have created together simply go down the drain.*

— *I'm afraid of being controlling, manipulative, unfair, egotistical, spiteful, weak and fragile like my mother and of consequently being accused by my children of not being a good mom.*

Next, Denise notes what expectations she has had of her husband and of herself in this situation.

— *I expected my husband to love me enough to understand my cry for help and that he would feel guilty if something should happen to me.*

— *I was hoping to be able to stop being so dependent on my husband so that I could finally be free to be myself instead of behaving like my mother.*

Now Denise is starting to recognize and feel that her fears for herself, as well as her expectations, are exactly the same as those experienced by her mother with her own spouse all her life. She takes the time needed to let this reality, which she had never seen before, really sink in.

Are you aware that having expectations of others and yourself indicates a lack of love and acceptance? It is your ego that is at work in all your expectations. They are not founded on reality. You are asking too much of yourself and also of others without giving yourself or others the right to have limits. The more we want to go beyond our limits, the more the harmful cells will go beyond their limits and the more serious the illness will be. The cells are but a reflection of what we create on the psychological level.

## You are the only one responsible for what you create

It is important to remember that cancer is not a virus coming from outside of us but something that comes, rather, from our own cells. Admitting and recognizing what she experiences in this situation as a result of her own fears and unrealistic expectations helps Denise to take responsibility. It is helping her moreover to see that this attitude does not meet her need and that she has attracted this type of situation in her life in order to become conscious.

## Triangle, mirror and reconciliation

The stage that comes next is very difficult for the ego. It is described as the *mirror* exercise. Indeed, every time you accuse another person of being anything whatsoever, it means that you are accusing yourself of the same thing and that this same person is also accusing you. It is the *triangle of life*. This triangle is also applicable to your experience of feelings and emotions and we all experience it to the same degree.

However, we should be aware that these accusations are, most of the time, not all related to the same behaviours. You can for example judge a person to be disrespectful when they are being impatient with you and that person can in turn judge you to be disrespectful when you are trying to control them or when you are interfering in their life.

**The only thing that is mirrored is what you ARE.**

The great law of attraction stipulates that we always attract what resonates with us. That is what explains why three people who, after meeting a fourth person for the first time, may each have a different opinion of that person. Nevertheless, all three of them were introduced to the person at the same time. Each of them perceived the new person through the lens of what they themselves are. They loved in the other person what they love in themselves and did not like what they do not yet accept in themselves.

Let us return to the example of Denise. To do the mirror exercise, she must note down the following sentences on paper, based on what she has already written, but beginning each sentence with *my mother* instead of with *I*:

– *My mother judged me and blamed me until today for being controlling, manipulative, unfair, egotistical, spiteful and fragile.*

– *My mother felt rejected, sad, angry, despairing, misunderstood, alone and isolated from me. She also felt that she did not have the right to exist as herself.*

– *My mother is afraid she will die if she continues to be dependent on her husband. She is also afraid that if she stops acting this way, she might decide to leave him. She is therefore afraid of losing the true love she experienced, of breaking up the family unit, of facing financial uncertainty, and seeing the cherished family life that they have created together simply go down the drain.*

It can be difficult to admit that the person with whom you have experienced a difficult situation has suffered as much as you have and has accused you of the same things of which you accuse them. This is why Denise has to take the necessary time to feel deeply that her mother suffered as much as she did and to the same degree. That is how she will be able to develop compassion for her. This exercise helps to open the heart, the way the person in the previous example could open the door that they had perceived as a wall.

When you succeed in truly feeling the pain of the other person, you will have completed the stage of reconciliation with that person. You will have a great sense of relief and you will not be able to resent that person any more.

## Forgiving yourself

We are now at the most important stage. But it is also the most difficult: forgiving oneself. Forgiving oneself is the greatest possible act of love toward oneself. However, it is imperative that you remember the resistance of your ego, for it is bound and determined to prevent you from going ahead with this type of action. You must on the other hand try to understand your ego. It knows that the more you love yourself, the less power it has over you. It experiences a visceral fear of losing its place and its authority over you. That's why you will hear several small inner voices telling you all sorts of things to prevent you from accepting the truth. We cannot blame our ego for acting this way, since when we decide to love rather than reject ourselves, our ego no longer comprehends anything and is totally confused.

**The ego has been so accustomed to you letting it decide for you, it is convinced that without it, you will suffer and possibly die.**

When you begin to accept yourself and love yourself, including those aspects of yourself with which you do not agree, it is an indication that you are reconnecting with your inner power. As you feed it less and less, your ego will start to shrink and will think that it is going to disappear for good. It is therefore important that, simultaneously with the acts of love you do for yourself, you reassure your ego that it will not disappear. Explain to it that the mental memory with which it was created will always be there, the only difference being that this memory will no longer have a hold over you.

Let us return to the example of Denise. To complete this stage, she must first of all accept herself and give herself permission to have resented her mother, to the point of having hated her at times. She needs to accept that it was this hatred that kept her in a state of constant fear and made her create unrealistic expectations.

Next, she must accept that she is what she accused her mother of being. This step will open up her heart permanently and optimally. Here is what this exercise looks like:

– *I admit that I too am at times controlling, manipulative, unfair, egotistical, spiteful and fragile. When I act that way it is because my wound of rejection is being strongly activated. I want so much not to behave this way that I choose to accuse others in order to avoid feeling how much I reject myself.*

This stage may take more time, but it is important that you go all the way with it. Your determination to want to reach self-acceptance will make all the difference in your life. You will then become conscious of the fact that when you believed it was only the *other* person you didn't accept, you were dealing with an illusion.

**In your life, others are only there to help you become conscious of what you do and do not accept in yourself.**

That is why the stage of reconciliation with the other, the stage where you accept that others are your mirror, needs to be completed before this final stage. Reconciliation helps you have compassion for the other person. It helps you start opening your heart.

Another reason why this stage is necessary is that it shows you how to proceed in the same fashion with yourself, how to have compassion for that part of you – the little inner child – that has been suffering for a long time. Always fearing rejection, it is still this part of you that reacts so strongly.

Since nothing can change or ever be transformed without first being accepted, this part of you must absolutely feel accepted and not rejected as if it was bad, undesirable, or a burden – to the point of wanting to cease to exist. The less accepted that part of you feels, the more it will resist and gain strength due to your ego. It will become more and more susceptible to rejection.

Have you ever tried to turn away a child who doesn't stop pestering you by telling them to go away, to go and play somewhere else? The more you turn them away, the harder they try to get your attention, even to the point of going overboard and playing nasty tricks, knowing perfectly well that their punishment will be all the greater for it. That's how you are treating those parts of yourself that you try to reject or fail to acknowledge. They finally want to take full control of you to prove they have a right to exist. This situation can, in the end, show up in the form of cancer cells.

The moment you accept the parts of yourself that are sometimes what you do not want to be, it's as if you were saying to that unruly child, *I know, sweetie, that you need attention. But I'm busy just now and I don't really have time. It has nothing to do with you if I feel stressed. It's that I simply do not know how to manage my time. I know that one day I will get there, but it's beyond my limits for now. If I don't take enough time for you, be assured that it has nothing to do with my love for you.*

On the other hand, one must not make promises one cannot keep. If for example Mom promises this child she will pay attention to him or her later and then doesn't, the child will not be able to respect her and will become even more unruly. All parents need to accept that they cannot always know how to handle the curves life throws them and at the same time deal with their children.

We often become parents before we have even finished being children ourselves. A future parent unfortunately doesn't have to obtain a diploma in parenting, as is required in many other occupations. Take consolation from the fact that your children are and always will be good instruments through whom you can become more conscious of what you do not accept in yourself.

I mentioned earlier that this stage was the most important because it is the one that starts the healing process in your body.

**Self-acceptance, which represents a great expression of love toward yourself, opens your spiritual heart.**

Is it possible that this opening up of the heart can have an instantaneous effect on your physical heart? Could it improve your blood and fill it with a healing balm, like a magnetism that circulates through your entire body and helps the cells to regenerate? This could be the phenomenon that explains why some people talk about a miracle.

I am so amazed by the way the physical body is created, and by its capacities, that I feel the heart possesses enormous powers. Have you ever asked yourself why this organ never suffers from cancer? The heart is in the centre of the body to remind you that when you come from your heart – from self-love and acceptance – you are centered.

To be centered means to be balanced. If you remain standing in the very centre of an enormous saucer turning really fast, you will not move, you will keep your balance. In such a situation, as soon as you try to move or try to go a little toward the edge, you will lose your balance and you will be projected outside the saucer. It is not by chance that Eastern medicine is so successful. Eastern philosophy is entirely based on balance in our life, in all fields.

## Connection with a parent

When the preceding stage of self-forgiveness has been completed, it is suggested that you make the connection with one or more situations from your childhood or adolescence during which you experienced those same things. I am not talking about the situation itself, but rather about what you experienced on the level of your emotions and accusations. It is very easy to make yourself believe that you no longer resent anyone with whom you experienced a problem, just as it is easy to make yourself believe that you accept yourself. This is another trick your ego plays on you. Remember that the ego is very shrewd about convincing people who are in their wound of rejection, because they are so susceptible to being in denial. In fact this is the greatest obstacle to fully achieving self-forgiveness.

Since it is harder to accept that we have resented, even hated, our parents, just managing to connect with these feelings and accusations is in itself a very precious step in the process toward complete forgiveness. It greatly increases your chances of healing. *Does there have to be a connection?* you will want to ask. Absolutely.

All emotional situations experienced as adults are nothing but repetitions of what happened during our childhood and adolescence. We are bound to live endless repetitions for as long as this type of situation is not experienced in acceptance. Unfortunately, people must come back life after life to experience the same thing, time and time again.

I have come to realize that the less we want to understand a message that is constantly being repeated to us, the more this message becomes important for helping the person see reality and move out of denial. It would explain why people bring a serious or even fatal illness upon themselves following a behaviour related to the wound of rejection. We often see others who experienced a similar trauma when they were young, but did not end up with such a serious illness. This would indicate that, in their case, it was a wound other than the wound of rejection that was activated.

**I know now that any serious physical or psychological illness is always related to the wound of rejection.**

Since cancer is directly linked to the wound of rejection and as this wound is experienced in relation to the parent of the same sex, Denise now asks herself the following question, repeating the same words as in the preceding stages:

— *In what situations did I accuse my mother of being ____ with my father or with me? In what situations did I feel ____ with fear for myself that_____?*

— *Is it possible that my mother judged me too, accused me of being the same thing in these situations, because of our common fear of_____?*

She then discovers several situations and every new awareness leads Denise deeper and deeper into her heart, where the light is. It is as if she found herself in a dark tunnel and every sincere answer that came in response to her questions brought her closer and closer to the bright light she perceived in the distance at the end of the tunnel. This light not only helps her to see reality, but to warm her spiritual heart. She is coming from her heart because she can feel suffering on both sides. She can no longer make accusations.

This warmth is also experienced throughout the body, a very welcome phenomenon for people suffering from rejection. These people are very sensitive to cold, often complaining that they feel chilly even when others around them say it is warm. They experience this sensation of cold because their great lack of self-love blocks the warmth.

**If you are often cold, it is your heart seeking the warmth of forgiveness and self-acceptance.**

**In other words, your heart wants you to love yourself as you are.**

## Sharing our experience

All that remains now is for Denise to go and express to her husband and share with him what she has discovered by completing the above stages. This will allow her to practise before undertaking this stage with her mother, who represents the ultimate test for becoming conscious that her process of forgiveness has truly been completed. I would remind you that your ego always resists more when you are dealing with a parent.

If, for example, Denise's ego were to raise all sorts of objections, including the ones given below, it would be a sign that she has not yet forgiven herself:

— *Don't go saying things like that to your husband and your mother, you know very well they will laugh at you, it won't make any sense to them.*

— *They've never read those kinds of books or done personal growth, they won't know what you're talking about.*

— *Your mother is already in poor health. Telling her things like this, especially that you hated her, is only going to make her feel worse. Better not to say anything.*

— *You don't need to go and see her, you know you have forgiven her, why bring up such painful memories?*

Another indication that you have not completely forgiven yourself is if we go to see our parent to ask for forgiveness for having judged and accused them and especially for having hated them. If you want another person to forgive you, it is a sign that you have not yet forgiven yourself. And if you tell the other person that you have forgiven them for having acted a certain way toward you, it shows that you still accuse them, that you judge their attitude as being unacceptable and that you do not want to see a recurrence.

Only self-forgiveness has the power to heal, not forgiveness of the other person. Self-forgiveness fills our blood with healing energy.

**No one has the power to forgive in someone else's place.**

To believe that we are so good that we can forgive another person the wrong they have done us is without a doubt one of the best ways to give great power to our ego. In the previous exercise, Denise does not forgive her mother for anything, because she is only showing compassion for her mother's suffering, which explains why she behaved that way. She accepts, observes and acknowledges the way a situation evolved. That way is neither good nor bad. It quite simply IS.

During this type of sharing, I suggest furthermore that you encourage your parent to talk, asking them when they experienced a situation involving the same accusations, emotions and fears for themselves with their parent of the same sex as you. Most of the time, the parent is able to go back to such a situation. It is surprising what a beautiful exchange there can be between a child and their parent when there is no accusation or judgment, but only compassion.

You will find at the end of this chapter Denise's testimonial sharing with us the happiness she felt when she contacted her mother following the forgiveness process she went through for her.

I suggest that you go and share what you have discovered. It is only by doing so that you can know if you truly accept yourself. If you are no longer judging yourself for having been mean and ungrateful toward your parent, if you have compassion for yourself and for the other, you will observe that it is much easier to share this discovery with this parent. The best test to know if you have taken your responsibility, and no longer resent this parent, is the gratitude you feel toward them. Instead of wanting to change them, you are grateful for what you have learned about yourself thanks to this parent.

## Summary of the seven stages

Here is a summary of the seven stages or steps of reconciliation and forgiveness that are suggested for dealing with any pain experienced with another person, in any situation.

1. Become aware of ACCUSATIONS made against the other person as well as the EMOTIONS experienced in the situation.

2. Take your RESPONSIBILITY knowing that it is your expectations of the other person as well as the fear you had for yourself that have attracted this situation.

3. RECONCILE yourself with the other person by accepting that they are accusing you of the same things, are experiencing the same fear for themselves and feel the same way you do in this situation.

4. FORGIVE yourself, showing compassion for the part of you that is suffering and is afraid.

5. Make the CONNECTION with the parent of the same sex as the person with whom you have experienced these emotions. With respect to cancer, it is always with the parent of the same sex as yourself.

6. DESIRE TO EXPRESS to the other person what you have experienced and what you are still experiencing. Take the time to prepare by picturing yourself doing this.

7. SEE THE PERSON CONCERNED and share with them what you have experienced and what you have learned about yourself thanks to this situation.

## Difficulty accepting oneself

If you realize that you find it difficult to forgive, and therefore, to go and share what you have experienced with your parent, accept yourself with this limit for now. It's because the suffering is too great and it is still impossible for you to forgive yourself. It is normal to seriously dislike oneself after becoming aware that the very behaviour we reproached one of our parents for, is the same behaviour we ourselves engaged in – toward them, toward others, but also toward ourselves.

Convinced that only other people are like that, our ego totally refuses to recognize this fact.

I want to reiterate that the ego is not capable of understanding or accepting any spiritual notion, for it is from mental energy that the ego was created. It can only think and reason, can only work with what the mental body has recorded in its memory. The spiritual dimension goes well beyond this; it is not limited to what can be proven or explained rationally. That is why the mental dimension – and hence, your ego – cannot understand anything that belongs to the spiritual dimension. The latter includes all notions of unconditional love, forgiveness, responsibility and acceptance.

Before you can share with your parent what you have experienced, take a few moments each day to visualize yourself actually conveying your experience while at the same time feeling the suffering that they feel just as intensely as you do. As your heart begins to open during these exercises, you will gradually succeed in truly accepting yourself and thus proceed to the other stages of true forgiveness. You will know you are ready to share your experience when you feel gratitude for this parent in this situation. Instead of wanting to change it, you will know that you needed this experience in order to know yourself better and love yourself more.

This reconciliation and forgiveness exercise is without a doubt the fastest and and most effective way to finally get a good picture of a situation, and of everyone involved in it, seen with the eyes of our heart. We can stop looking at the situation with blinkers on - the blinkers of our ego - which enormously restrict our vision of people and of things.

**Only after you have accepted it with your heart, can you manifest true understanding of any situation. And this is possible only when you take your responsibility.**

As you can observe, each step brings you further and further into your heart and into true love. It is only in the fourth step – the one involving self-forgiveness – that you find yourself back in the light which alone has the great power of healing. All that is left for you to do is allow the energy emanating from your divine heart to do the work it needs to do in your body. The last three steps are very important as a verification of whether the stage of self-forgiveness has really been completed.

## Is healing possible for everyone?

It is impossible to state that a person who has succeeded in forgiving themselves will automatically heal. It is true that I have witnessed countless healings over the last thirty years and am therefore in a position to help people have hope.

I have on the other hand known people who have really forgiven themselves and who nevertheless succumbed to death, but feeling at peace with themselves. I conclude that they died healed, for true healing must take place beyond the physical world. Generally speaking, the body reflects what is happening on the psychological level. But if our physical and psychological suffering have been going on for too long, it is possible that the physical body no longer has the necessary strength to reverse the process and return to its state of natural health. Could it be, then, that certain souls, knowing they have reached their goal of self-forgiveness, choose to return to the world of the soul? Who knows? It's their life, their choice.

I have also witnessed people who did not reach the point of being able to forgive themselves and who died taking with them all the pain caused by the hatred or bitterness that inhabited them. These people will however be able to continue their process of forgiveness in another life more peacefully if they give themselves permission now to have limits and accept their inability to attain their goal at this time.

Whether a person's life is extended or not, the most important thing is that the true forgiveness that they have initiated has contributed to the healing of their soul, which will make a big difference for them in the world of the soul and in their next life.

**To heal is to release everything that blocks our energy. To heal is to regain our lost freedom.**

In summary, anyone who wants to help a sick person must do so not in order to try and heal them physically, but rather in order to offer support on the level of the soul.

I mentioned in the second chapter that, with the present energy of the Age of Aquarius, everything is accelerated. This energy can be used to accelerate illness or the harmful effects of cancer. But it may also and especially be used to accelerate the process of healing.

I am thinking here of two different cases. The first is that of a man around forty years of age who was dealing with cancer. Let's call him Robert. I can't remember where or how this cancer started but when I met him at one of my workshops, his right side at waist level was full of cancer. He appeared to be suffering enormously. He could neither sit nor sleep comfortably except in one particular chair. Furthermore, he always came to the workshops with another person who took care of transporting that chair.

Robert had chosen to come and settle in Quebec, having left France to escape his father of whom he was very much afraid. His father had decided that his son was going to be a great athlete to make up for the fact that he himself had not been able to realize such a dream. His father, having had a domineering father himself, had become a prosperous businessman in the hope that it would earn him his father's respect.

Robert emulated this behaviour and did everything he could so his dad would love him. He forced himself to do a lot of physical training, he practised several different sports. But despite all his efforts, his dad never seemed satisfied. His dad never took the trouble to congratulate his son on his successes, yet never missed an opportunity to criticize him at the slightest slipup.

One day Robert had had enough. He left home, got married and had four children. In the meantime, his father continued to hassle him, criticize him and disagree with all his choices. That's when he decided to come to live in Quebec. The year after the move, Robert began to get sick and learned afterwards that he had cancer. When his father found out, he insisted Robert approach a well-known American specialist for treatment and was prepared to foot the enormous bill if he would go ahead with it. He called Robert repeatedly to try and get him to listen to reason.

Still reacting against his father, Robert decided to do just the opposite. He decided he wouldn't have any doctor look after him and would invest his energy instead in personal growth.

My initial advice to him was however to consider getting help from the medical profession because his case was very serious. Often accompanying him to the workshops, his wife was of the same opinion as I was. When I saw that he vehemently opposed the idea, I told myself that if at least he could make a truce with his father and with himself, using the various stages of forgiveness, he could only benefit.

Robert sincerely wanted to achieve reconciliation with his father, but his wound of rejection was such that he couldn't manage it. His cancer appeared just around the time when he noticed he was becoming like his father, even while living far away from him. For instance, he was becoming more and more demanding toward his sons and even ended up striking them when they didn't listen to him. Afterwards he would go and hide in the basement of the house, shedding hot tears and criticizing himself for being no better than his father. He was nevertheless convinced that by living far away from his father, he would not experience this type of anger.

Robert took part in several workshops, listened carefully and even reached a point where he felt that his father loved him in his way and didn't know any other way to love him, because he was imitating the little love he himself had received. However, unfortunately, he never managed to forgive himself for having hated his father so much and for having acted like his father, with the result that his sons hated him too. He died in this state, but with nevertheless the consolation of having had the sincere desire to achieve reconciliation. In the end, his pain proved to be too intense for this to be possible in this life.

The other case that speaks to me is this friend, whom I'll call Normand, whom I saw at the hospital a few weeks before his death and who, in the space of a few hours, understood everything and felt the rejection experienced with his dad. He had never realized the pain he had gone through with his father, for his father had him placed in a psychiatric institution when Normand was just a little boy. He was afterwards raised by his mother and had in fact hardly known his father. Normand was a very rigid kind of person and it was easy to see in his body his great wounds of rejection and injustice.

As he opened up and spoke of his childhood and as he was able to feel more and more everything that he had experienced over all these years, but had repressed, I could feel what was happening inside him. I could perceive in his eyes all the transformations that little by little were taking place in him. It was a very beautiful experience both for him and for me and we both wept tears of happiness. I could feel the compassion he had for his father and for himself.

Before leaving him that evening, Normand admitted to me that he felt his body to be so exhausted that it was now the same to him whether he would live or die. I felt reassured however by the look in his eyes which shone with peace and happiness. I even remember thinking to myself how very much the eyes are the window of the soul. I knew then that he was truly healed, even if he should choose not to live any longer. I was not surprised to learn of his death a few weeks later.

What is most important in Normand's case is that he died with peace in his heart and that he succeeded in experiencing his father's pain as well as his own. He had been suffering for a long time, hardly eating. He hadn't told anyone, wanting to fight this illness on his own. He had to see his body reach its limit before he decided to go and see a doctor. When the time comes for Normand to return in another, healthy, body, he will not have to relive this same experience and will be able to continue to move forward on the journey of his soul.

## Breaking free

As long as you continue to bear a grudge against another person, you remain a prisoner. It's as if you were constantly joined to that other person by a rope. You need to understand that this rope was created with one of your parents when you were very young. The stronger the grudge and the greater the hatred, the thicker the rope and the harder it is to break it. The thickness of the rope represents the degree of the suffering experienced with this parent. Each time another person makes you relive this same pain, you feel this same rope imprisoning you and blocking the energy that wants to flow freely in your body.

This is why so many people who experience not only grudges but also hatred feel imprisoned by thick ropes. Feeling more and more powerless, they finally end up creating serious illnesses. Each of these illnesses is the reflection of the energy blockage caused by the ropes.

I regularly hear people say that they would not under any circumstances forgive the person who they believe did them so much harm. It is the other person who should be coming to them to ask for forgiveness. You would be right to suspect that this kind of talk comes from their ego and not their heart. Indeed, the ego knows that we never attract a situation or a person that does not resonate with us. EVERYTHING ORIGINATES FROM WITHIN.

These people think that by refusing to see or speak to the other person, they are punishing them and they themselves will be freeer. In the previous example it was clear that Robert continued to suffer mightily despite having fled to Canada to avoid seeing or hearing his father anymore. The rope created by his hatred so imprisoned him that he could not break free of it. He thought he could liberate himself from a constraint by changing his physical context but had to face the truth that nothing in his life had changed because he had not undergone any inner transformation.

A woman told me once that she hated her mother-in-law so much that she thought about it incessantly and would even wake up at night with hateful thoughts of her. At the time I met her, the woman in question was facing her third bout of cancer. She came to one of our *Listen to Your Body* workshops and quickly realized that what we teach is reconciliation and self-forgiveness. She then let us know in no uncertain terms, *I shall never be able to forgive that horrible woman, after everything she has done to me. If you cannot advocate other methods of healing for me, I will not be coming back*.

I then told her that she was not obliged to do this exercise at this time and that it would even be preferable that she give herself more time so her chances of succeeding later would be better. Adamantly opposed to the idea of reconciliation with her mother-in-law, she insisted other methods be suggested to her, on the spot. I invited her to pursue private counselling. She replied that she had been in therapy for years and nothing had changed. After that exchange, I never saw the poor woman again. Clearly, she was suffering terribly.

In my experience, the stages of reconciliation and self-forgiveness are the fastest and most efficient way to shrink the thickness of the rope which will finally break in due course. That will spell true freedom for both parties involved.

If people only realized how much energy it takes to maintain this hatred, and thereby create this kind of rope, they would be in more of a hurry to break free of it as quickly as possible in order to finally regain their natural energy and thus be able to create anything they want in life.

If you are maintaining this kind of hatred, you will know exactly what I am talking about, because you must very often feel tired for no apparent reason. And that's perfectly normal. And it is also possible to observe that people who are struggling with a major wound of rejection can eat a huge amount of food without ever gaining weight because the energy from the food is trying to make up for all the energy spent on maintaining the hatred.

Even if sometimes it takes several years, what sweet victory when the rope is broken and freedom is finally regained. It is my heartfelt wish that this great happiness should be experienced by everyone. **I remind you that this real forgiveness can only occur when you forgive yourself for being like the person against whom you bear a grudge or that you hate.**

In conclusion, know that real forgiveness has the power to restore the natural flow of energy throughout the body. When this occurs, the energy in your body leads you toward your life plan, whether it be to live or to die. The essential thing is that you should be at peace with yourself and able to attract to yourself a beautiful life or a magnificent transition to the hereafter.

To end this chapter, I would like to offer the testimony of Denise, who kindly agreed to describe in writing all the stages of the forgiveness process that she went through with her mother and with herself.

## Testimony of Denise

*Dear readers,*

*At Lise Bourbeau's request, I am sharing my story with you, which includes my journey following the news of my breast cancer in 2012. Thanks to Lise's marvellous therapeutic skills, I was able to deeply change my way of being and thinking.*

*Faced with a cancer diagnosis, I knew that my body was giving me a powerful message and that I needed to silence my ego and let my feelings speak and above all, listen to them without filtering them, listen with compassion toward myself.*

*There were two important exchanges with LIse that played a decisive role in my healing from cancer. The first exchange allowed me to define the events that lay at the root of this cancer, which were a result of the conflictual relationship I had with my mom. The second exchange was a "revelation" and a "liberation" so powerful that I will never forget the incredible physical sensation I felt in my heart once I realized and accepted, with full awareness, my share of responsibility in the conflict that had existed between my mother and myself ever since I was a child.*

*From that instant, I knew that I was on the path to being healed, not just physically, but also psychologically and spiritually. When my eyes met LIse's, I understood that she too felt that certainty. It was March 19, 2013.*

*I had not been in touch with my mother for five years (I live in Quebec and she lives in France) and didn't know how to approach the forgiveness stage with her. I addressed the Divine and waited for a sign, an opportunity. On March 21 – two days later –, I finally received the sign I had been waiting for. The day before my birthday and after years of silence, an email from my mother wishing me a happy birthday and asking me how I was doing! The door to the forgiveness stage had just been opened...*

*So I called my mother to tell her my news and let her know about the diagnosis of breast cancer, which she knew nothing of. As if by magic, I no longer felt in me any negative emotional charge toward her when speaking with her. In fact this exchange just confirmed that I was no longer afraid of being rejected by my mother while we were talking. And furthermore, that first conversation went on a very long time.*

*I then shared with her all the stages of my story, then the stages of forgiveness. It was done with gentleness. We listened to each other with honesty, without judgment. It was suddenly so easy. Without apprehension, I told her about all the sadness, the pain caused by her insistence that her children call her Kitty instead of mom from the time they could talk. I was able to be open even though I knew I was broaching a sensitive topic for her. By sharing my experience with her, I felt inside myself that I no longer needed for her to behave in any particular way in order to feel comfortable.*

*Her listening, her new openness, nevertheless allowed me to be real. I had never been able to exchange like this with her before, and the most surprising thing for me was that I spoke with her as if I had seen her just the day before. The past, the conflicts no longer had any hold over our "new" relationship.*

*At the conclusion of that call, I became filled with a deep sense of peace and love. Since that time, we call each other regularly. A holistic medicine enthusiast, my mother gives me wonderful advice, which I apply and find very effective for my health. We speak openly for hours, feeling close, something we had never enjoyed before. Moreover, when she sends me an email, she signs mom and not Kitty the way she used to, even though I have told her that I am now comfortable calling her Kitty. I found my mom again, a mom I thought I had lost. And I love her as she is.*

*Besides restoring my relationship with my mother, this cancer also allowed me to regain my affective independence from my spouse. The wound of rejection from which I had suffered since childhood had made me dependent on him affectively and dependent on some of his addictions. I was so afraid of losing his love and of not being able to be "on his wave length" that I "copied" in part some of his behaviours in order to please him.*

*Thanks to the realization I had during my second meeting with LIse, I was able to make the connection between my wound of rejection and this affective dependence. I understood that I had to leave him free to be himself without trying to change him. I was the one who had to change by respecting my basic needs and altering the belief that I would lose him if I did not act in accordance with his expectations or what I thought were his expectations of me.*

*Gradually, I detached myself emotionally from my husband and the "harmful" behaviours I associated with him. To do this, the exercise of conscious letting go helped me a lot. There were a lot of clashes between us at first, but these soon became less frequent. My husband is also a fan of Listen to Your Body teaching and understood the issues, the reasons for my actions.*

*Of his own accord, he also undertook personal growth work at the same time as me, resulting in significant improvement in dealing with his addiction problems. This was achieved in a few weeks and we are now more united than ever!*

*This cancer has been for me a journey of initiation. I had intellectualized about many "therapeutic concepts" such as forgiveness, letting go, acceptance, unconditional love, etc. I talked about them a lot and in a very positive way because I did believe in them, but it remained at the intellectual level. It was the cancer that allowed me to really "integrate" these ideas. I experienced them in "my gut", for good, because I have finally given myself permission to feel the rejection I went through with my mother. It was sometimes painful but ever so freeing, for my mother was merely the reflection I needed. I have understood the message and will never forget it.*

*I continue to learn and to co-create with the Divine in me and around me, in harmony and in unity and with much compassion when sometimes I still stray from the path toward loving myself.*

# Chapter Seven

## The importance of taking a decision

In the preceding chapter, I explained the importance of forgiving yourself in order to begin the healing process – both physical and psychological. There is another factor that is just as important and that is the WILL TO LIVE. To be more precise, it is not enough only to "not want to die," if you are among those who have cancer or are afraid of a relapse. The example of Richard in Chapter Five shows clearly the very positive effect his "will to live" had on him.

So many people, after they learn they have cancer, undertake a series of actions because they don't want to die. They change their diet, alter their lifestyle, quit smoking, stop drinking, go to bed earlier, get more physical exercise, see healing practitioners and therapists... If all these actions are carried out for the purpose of NOT dying and NOT having cancer any more, the intention is not the right one.

Remember that the subconscious works only with the images that our thoughts or words evoke. All the sentences spoken or thought in the negative form, with the word NOT, contribute to increasing what you do not want. Your subconscious, rather than picturing you as healed, pictures you only in images associated with the words you use – even if they represent what you do not want – like "die" and "cancer".

You may ask, *Why would you try and persuade me to want to live when I have just found out that I am suffering from a fatal illness?* The best path is to take the decision to live. The words I AM DECIDING TO LIVE, I WANT TO LIVE must become louder than your fear of dying.

To be able to take this kind of decision, you must first of all have a good reason to live. What do you want for yourself in this life? The following question can definitely help you to come up with the answer.

**If all circumstances were perfect, that is, if you had the time, the health and the money required, and your needs were accepted by those around you, what would you want?**

I would strongly encourage you to sit down in a quiet place and take the time to note as many desires as possible. Then, add beside each one what these desires can help you to BE in your life. For example: *I want to stop working in order to devote myself to painting, I want to develop my artistic talents.* This desire may particularly help you to *be enthusiastic, excited, joyful, creative, etc*. If you have difficulty discoving the "to be" part, you can use the following interrogative sentence: *This desire helps me to feel how?* By adding what a desire will help you to "be," you discover what your soul needs.

The next stage is to note the intensity of each of these needs on a scale of 1 to 10, 10 being a significant manifestation. It is interesting to discover or note that the fear of dying is sometimes necessary in order to remember all the desires and needs that we have set aside over time. Don't forget, therefore, to thank this fear for helping you to become aware of them.

## The right to live for oneself

If you say, *I want to live to look after my four-year-old daughter; I want to help her grow up, marry and have children,* then when you realize that this child is more important than you at this time, welcome this desire. But I want to remind you that you exist and live on this Earth uniquely for yourself. This wish is however very legitimate and can furthermore give you the strength to live longer. But to ensure true transformation or a stronger immune system, I suggest taking this wish a step further. Observe and sense deeply inside yourself what feeling this wish makes you experience. How does this desire, when it manifests itself, help you to be and help you to know yourself?

First of all, rest assured, you have the right to live for yourself and that should be your greatest goal in life. It is not selfish to think that way, it's loving yourself. Let me give you the definition of the word *selfish*, something I am obliged to do in all my books, talks and workshops. Why? Because most people have trouble thinking of themselves before they think of others, because they think that's selfish. I have furthermore observed that that same belief resides in every country where I have taught so far. What a mistaken definition of a word, developed over several lifetimes!

**To be selfish is to want the other person to look after your needs before their own. To love yourself is to look after your own needs before the needs of others.**

As you can see, wanting to live for yourself is the opposite of selfishness. In fact, it is a true expression of love for yourself. When I travel by plane, the flight attendants always advise passengers to make sure they have put on their own oxygen mask securely before trying to help another person (a child, their spouse, etc.). They obviously understand that *true charity begins at home*.

It is very likely that if you are the type of person who believes they are responsible for the happiness of others, you will see this notion as being very egotistical. I assure you that it is not. Every soul is on this Earth for its own development and not for the development of others. Every soul needs to be surrounded by loved ones to become conscious of the work they need to do for their own development.

That is why you must not insist on wanting to live just for another person or other people. That kind of decision can only attract a good deal of emotion later on. For example, I can easily imagine what might happen to the mom who chose to want to live only for her daughter, should her daughter choose a life path in life that goes totally against the mother's expectation. The mother will surely say to herself, and perhaps even to her daughter or other people, *I fought to stay alive for her sake and this is how she repays me, this is all I mean to her. What an ungrateful daughter.*

The big decision to live will however give you the strength to make some favorable changes in your life, even if it's frightening. No matter how great your desire to live, there will probably be fears that come to plague you all the same. When they manifest, be sure to welcome them for they are human and completely normal. Tell the little voices inside you that it is normal that they should try to frighten you and think they are helping you that way.

In fact, they are convinced it might be preferable for you to die instead of continuing to suffer because of the rejection that you feel and the lack of love you experience. Tell them quite simply that you have decided to live and that you are ready to assume the consequences of your decision.

You need to know that these fears also help you to develop the courage you need in order to take action. Become aware that the harmful mutating cells that are circulating in your body are present there in order to draw your attention to the fact that your soul wants to mutate, which according to the dictionary means to change by virtue of receiving a new assignment. Rest assured that your soul is ready for this change.

This great desire to live will also help you to get a second wind, like an athlete who feels they can't go any further, who thinks they have no strength left, but whose determination to want to reach their goal is so great that they are filled with a second wind that may even help them exceed all their previous levels of performance. This type of phenomenon cannot be explained scientifically because that new strength comes from beyond our physical, emotional and mental capacities. It comes from our great inner power. This reminds me of the story about the mother who lifted a truck to free her child's leg which was pinned underneath it.

That decision to live explains furthermore why certain people, after many years of living in concentration camps or dismal prisons, succeed in rising above their experience, or why others finding themselves alone at sea, hanging on to a piece of wood after a shipwreck, manage to survive. These accounts are often considered to be real miracles.

It is indeed said, *Where there is hope, there is life*. We can compare hope to the light in the distance, at the end of the tunnel. The person who holds on to this hope never stops looking at that light. They look ahead of them. If they don't, if they look back, they risk staying stuck in the past, forgetting that light, forgetting the life awaiting them at the tunnel's exit.

Knowing that despair accelerates the proliferation of harmful cells threefold – according to statistics – gives us a good idea of the power hope can awaken. Whether we despair or are hopeful, it is our inner power that is at work, this power being influenced by whether or not we take the decision to want to live.

**The question to ask yourself is: Do I want to use my power to live or to die?**

## The importance of acceptance

I want to come back again to the importance of acceptance as a way to ensure you feel greater certainty about your decision to live. What is it you need to accept? Accept that it is your fear of rejection that attracted this cancer. When I say illness is an expression of what is happening within you, it doesn't mean you are guilty of having created the illness.

I especially want you to know that if your thoughts have the power to block energy from circulating freely in your body, they equally have the power to get that energy flowing again, with the result that the illness process will be reversed so that the healing process can begin. By taking responsibility for your illness, you are also getting back in touch with your immense power to create.

Please note that cancer is definitely not a punishment from GOD. It is, rather, the opposite. It is an indication that you have forgotten your inner GOD. You have forgotten:

- hat being GOD means you are on this Earth to learn to love yourself completely and unconditionally;
- that your inner GOD wants to draw your attention to the fact that you are lacking in love for your self;
- that all your experiences are nothing more than a variety of experiences to help you become conscious of what you still need to do;
- that you are not a worthless person, that you have a right to exist;
- that even if you have suffered enough, to the point where you feel hate, it is simply an indication of your great need for love in your life.

GOD is the energy that pulses through everything that is alive. God is not an entity that enjoys choosing to punish or reward anyone whomsoever. We all represent this immense divine energy that wishes only to live, and is willing to learn through our experiences as a human being. Accordingly, we will all eventually end up living in a way that is more intelligent and more beneficial for us.

It is important therefore not to believe that you are the only person who experiences what you are going through. Everyone dealing with this illness finds it very difficult, but it is only the outer expression of what is going on inside them that is different.

## Miracles

One of the ways this acceptance changes a person's life is that they begin to attract miracles of all kinds. I have witnessed so many miracles in my life that it is easy for me to state that it is our self-acceptance, our love for ourself and the decisions we take that are responsible for our healing. At *Listen to Your Body*, we have gathered thousands of testimonies to this effect for conditions ranging from simple ailments to more serious illnesses, of a physical as well as a psychological nature.

WHAT IS A MIRACLE? According to the dictionary, a miracle designates *a fact that is extraordinary, positive and scientifically inexplicable*. It is mostly seen as a supernatural phenomenon attributed to a divine power, carried out either directly by this divinity or indirectly through one of its intermediaries.

Miracles are always experienced after a person has taken a firm decision that has helped them connect with their divine power. A miracle never comes from outside of us, but quite definitely from inside. Only those who refuse to accept their own divine power will attribute the miracle to heavenly intervention.

Usually when people talk about miracles, it is in relation to the physical body, but miracles happen on all levels. For example, a young man arrives in a foreign country whose language he has never heard before and finds that in just two weeks, he is speaking the language fluently.

The way I understand it, a miracle designates an event that happens spontaneously, rather than through a process of months or years. This phenomenon can only take place when the person has strong certainty and unwavering faith. The story I quoted before about one of my aunts who was dying of a cancer that had spread throughout her body and was then healed is a good example. She had been confined to her bed ever since her discharge from hospital but decided one day, in her husband's absence, to get up, get dressed and take the bus to Ste-Anne-de-Beaupré, a well-known pilgrimage site in Quebec. She left her husband a note instructing him not to look for her and that she had left to make a novena.

After her return nine days later, my aunt improved steadily. Six months later and following the required examinations by her doctor, it was reported to her that there was no longer any trace of cancer in her body. Just the fact of going alone to Quebec on the bus, a trip that took several hours, was already a miracle in itself. In fact, my aunt had truly taken the decision to live. She died forty years later from a heart problem.

Like many others, you may think that it is not her doing that this miracle happened, but rather the intervention of a divine power. That's fine. But once we become aware that all of us are this divine energy, it is not hard to see that we all have enough power to heal ourselves. It all depends on whether we connect to this energy within ourselves or not.

Another kind of miracle I have often witnessed during workshops or private sessions is when in response to a question, the client touches on something very important after their heart has opened. In fact, all the *Listen to Your Body* methods are deliberately based on questions. That way, it is up to the client to find the answers themselves. That is a much more effective approach than if we ourselves were to tell them the cause of their problem. It is more of an experiential method than a didactic one.

I call these experiences *moments of grace*, for the client as well as the facilitator or therapist. In my case, the strong feeling that the person has just taken a major decision, even if they are not yet conscious of it, is so powerful that it sends a shiver through my body and my head, and often tears come to my eyes. It is a moment when I feel that the person has just effected a major turnaround in their life, accepts what has been and becomes open to orienting themselves toward what they want to see in the future. Healing is under way.

I have also several times been the witness of health problems being healed spontaneously. Within a few minutes of these moments of grace, the person claims they are no longer in pain. If I happen to see them again later, they tell me that the problem never returned. I always recommend in such cases that they go back to their doctor to have the healing confirmed.

It is possible on the other hand that the healing has taken place only on the mental level, that the person was healed by the power of their will and that they did not really go through the stages of acceptance and self-forgiveness. If this is the case, there is a strong possibility that the same health problem will reappear later. This often occurs through different forms of cancer. Could this be why many doctors do not want to come out and say that the person is healed, preferring to tell them that the cancer is just in remission? It is only through the ability to feel deeply that we can know for certain whether we are healed, whether the necessary soul work has been done.

But how can these types of miracles be explained? Is it possible to consider that all our feelings and emotions are carried through our system in our blood, that as soon as there is a major change in what we feel, there is a similar change in the quality of our blood? I am convinced that love generates a great deal of magnetism, of healing power in our blood flow. Our cellular memories too are all carried in our blood. Accordingly as we make peace with others and with ourselves, we change our memory for the better. We become aware that the people we hated are not what we thought.

How many times have I not heard people tell me, now that they perceive their parents with the eyes of their heart, that they realize they loved them much more than they thought. They even start to remember scenes from the past that confirm this new perception.

**The present moment is changing our past and our future in the same degree.**

I believe, furthermore, that it is not important to try to understand the phenomenon of healing any more than we need to try to obtain proof. Why? Because things that are of a spiritual nature, things that come from beyond the mental dimension, cannot be understood on the mental level. That reminds me of a little story I heard several years ago.

A large group of lepers lived on an island. One day they saw a boat being rowed up to the shore and a man got out. He gathered all the lepers together and announced that he had discovered a remedy that could heal them. He brought out a box filled with little jars and he explained what the medication was and the benefits it offered. Then he said to them, *The only condition of your healing is that you remember EXACTLY how to take these potions and follow the directions perfectly.*

The man then indicated how they should take a certain amount the first three days, then stop for a certain period, resume for two days, and so forth, until they finished the medication. He made them repeat all that he said because no one had anything to write with.

The man returned to his boat and the group began to take the medication. But on the second day already, each of them began to doubt the man's remarks and to ask themselves a lot of questions, stubbornly resisting his claims about what was in the medication and its benefits. They wondered particularly whether the man was really a doctor and where he came from. They were so preoccupied with wanting to understand everything that they forgot how they were supposed to take it. You know how the story ends. No one was healed.

That was just to illustrate that if you do not understand how a miracle was possible, accept it for the time being. Maybe one day you will understand it, if your soul expresses the need.

## The wrong way to listen to your needs

There are a lot of people who unconsciously hold the belief that their cancer will enable them to listen to their needs. How is this possible? So far, we have seen that the profile of a person with cancer usually shows someone inclined to listen to the needs of others before their own. It is therefore quite common for this type of person to hope their cancer will grant them permissions they did not dare grant themselves when they were in good health.

You have to admit that a sick person gets a lot more attention than someone who is well. The sick person feels entitled to rest, to say no to certain requests, even though fewer requests are made of a sick person. They furthermore have permission to work less and even to take paid sick leave. In the case of the mother of a family, it is others who will now look after her, the opposite of the usual scenario.

To know whether this applies to you, check your reaction when someone refuses to look after you when you are sick. Do you think that because you have cancer or another illness, your family and friends must set aside their own needs to focus solely on yours? Do you believe that it is now their turn to do what you have always done? You need to know that this kind of attitude does nothing but encourage irresponsibility and feelings of guilt.

If you recognize yourself in this attitude, be aware that it is your ego trying to play a trick on you. If you do fall into this trap, you are contributing to developing a victim mentality, and then the cost of learning to listen to your own needs becomes much too high. The message here is rather to learn to give yourself all these permissions without having to get sick first. You are the only one who can listen to your real needs. Others cannot do this for you. Otherwise, you will want to remain ill, thereby encouraging the cancer to take a long time to stabilize. And even if you were completely healed of it, you risk attracting a relapse or another illness.

## The right to want to die

Other people are convinced they just don't have the strength to go on living and they want, no matter what, to be done with life. This is often true in the cases of rapidly advancing cancer. Since what is at issue here is YOUR life, YOUR body and YOUR decision, you certainly have the right to want to die, even should you be aware that your family and friends will inevitably be affected. You are not accountable to anyone, you are the only person responsible for your life.

I want to remind you that the reaction of your family and friends is a good indicator of your own acceptance of your choice. If you feel guilty for wanting to stop living badly enough to be willing to leave your loved ones, they will certainly not accept your choice. They will reproach you and will want to convince you of the opposite with the same intensity with which you judge and accuse yourself.

I would suggest at this point that you draw up a list of all your reasons for wanting to die, just like you would do for wanting to live. People who attract cancer into their life have, it seems, the unconscious desire to die. It is as if they believed that this kind of solution would make it easier to face a situation that is just too difficult to go through. I want to emphasize that I said *an unconscious desire*, as that is the most common, but it is not always the case. Indeed, several of these people have admitted to me that they entertained the thought of death at one time or another.

When you have finished your list, you can let your family and friends know what your decision is and you can give yourself the right to take that decision – if you consider it would be preferable to die. That doesn't necessarily mean that's what will happen. There are so many surprising things that can still happen after you have accepted your decision. Remember that the Universe knows your needs even better than you do. You might think that your decision really comes from the deepest part of you, but it could instead be your ego that has succeeded in influencing you without you realizing it.

And that is the reason I suggest to everyone that they make a list with the reasons why they want to live as well as the reasons why they want to die. By making both lists, you can feel certain that the final decision you make really comes from you.

## Don't wait until you are well in order to live

When someone shares with me the news that they have cancer and I then ask how they feel and what decision they have made, they often tell me they have decided they want to live and that as soon as they are better, they will do this, they will do that. I then remind them that their decision does not appear to be solidly rooted in them yet. They must DECIDE TO LIVE NOW. Live as if they did not have this sword of Damocles hanging over them.

Others stay on guard, not really listening to their needs, even after receiving their doctor's confirmation that the cancer has disappeared *for now*. These people continue living in fear of the word *relapse*, which they almost certainly hear as an imminent death sentence. Having also been told that a returning cancer is more aggressive in most people, they carry this fear inside them constantly.

If you ever feel troubled by this fear, welcome it and tell your ego that you understand that it believes it is helping you by scaring you, but that you have nonetheless decided to live and are ready to assume the consequences of your decision, even if things don't always go as you would wish and even if your wound of rejection is not yet healed. Take the time to explain to your ego the reasons why you want to live. It might tell you you'll never succeed, but remember that it is basing itself solely on things learned and experienced in the past.

# Chapter Eight

## How to deal with cancer in a loved one

Some people find it harder to receive the news that a friend or family member has cancer, as if it involved them personally. They think, furthermore, that they need to be stronger if they are to be able to handle it. Feeling very close, they experience great emotional upheaval most of the time at the idea of losing this person, in addition to feeling everything that this person is going through.

The most difficult cancer to accept in another person is generally cancer in a child. People say things like:

— *It's not fair. He has barely begun his life!*

— *Why did my child die of cancer when my grandfather who is so old and sick is still living? Where does the power to decide come from?*

— *Why has my teenager been stricken with cancer when she had such plans for her future? Why doesn't it happen to the aimless ones, the drifters, the loafers, the drug addicts?*

— *I don't understand how you can say it's an illness of repressed emotions, when my son was the very picture of joie de vivre. He was a real live wire and the most outgoing one in the family.*

— *How can you say that the wound of rejection is at the root of cancer when we so longed for this child of ours?*

The wound of rejection has nothing to do with whether a child is wanted or not. In the example of Denise, which I used to explain reconciliation and self-forgiveness, she was the eldest child and very much a wanted child. That did not prevent her from feeling rejected when, for instance, her mother wished to be called *Kitty* or controlled her every move and Denise could never feel free, and so forth.

I know with certainty that her mother was convinced she was a good mother, that she sincerely believed that the way she treated her daughter was a way of showing her love. Perhaps she believed that having her three children call her *Kitty* would help them see her more as a friend than a mom. It is very likely that she herself would have liked her mother to be her friend.

How could someone feel rejected then? Because we are born with this wound and it is experienced in differing degrees by each of us. Moreover, when we create a hard shell around us in order not to feel it (the shell of the wound of injustice, called the *rigid* mask), we ensure that we won't feel anything and will repress it all, which then contributes to experiencing everything alone, and that isolation is a common factor with all cancers.

The other important factor, based on my observations, is the effect of several accumulated lives. How can I be so sure of this? It was after hundreds of private regression sessions – going back to the fetal stage and to previous lives – with all kinds of people, that I was able to establish the influence of unsettled matters from previous lives on this present life. In fact, we arrive on Earth with a life plan, that is to say, with a very specific purpose, to help our soul return to the light.

One can compare all the lives of a soul to all the days of a life on Earth. If for example, a friend or family member was very violent toward you and you shouted angrily that you never wanted to see him or her again, it is not because the next day is a new day that the matter is settled. During all the days, months or years that follow, that problem will continue to haunt you and make you feel so bad that one day you will want to find a way to deal with it in order to feel better. The pain experienced takes up more and more room whether you are conscious of it or not. This pain creates an energy blockage in you and ends up manifesting itself in the form of illness.

As I have pointed out a number of times in this book, we can live in peace and serenity only when we take responsibility for everything that happens to us and accept people and situations, which means refraining from any judgment as to whether they are good or bad, and only welcoming the situation or the person.

There is a high risk of cancer among individuals who are born into a family where the parent of the same sex is someone with whom they have already lived other lives but with whom acceptance of self and acceptance of the other were not achieved. No matter what the attitude of this parent, the child will invariably feel rejected. The child recognizes this soul from the moment of birth, but does so unconsciously. During a regression session, it will often happen that, upon seeing their parent of the same sex, the individual says, *Oh no, not him again* or *not her again!* But then it is quickly forgotten. We are not psychologically stable enough to remember our past lives or most of our early childhood memories. Actually, we think we could not handle the suffering that the accompanying sense of rejection would evoke.

So, why then would cancer strike a very young child? With the Age of Aquarius, everything is very much accelerated. Is it possible then that the soul of this child wished to deal just with one specific thing and that once it was accomplished, it chose this way to leave? I have often observed this phenomenon in children with leukemia. So many parents have shared with me that their child seemed very serene, spoke about their death with ease and acceptance and helped the rest of the family to accept it.

Many families with children who have leukemia have furthermore learned great lessons about life thanks to this experience. There are others who on the other hand, continue to rail against the injustice of it for many years, unable to accept the death of their child. These people have not learned that no one belongs to anyone, that we have all been attracted in order to be part of the same family because we all need one another.

Remember that you are here FOR YOU and that everyone around you is there only to help you to know yourself and help you to practise unconditional love.

## Fear or solace?

I know it is totally normal to feel shock upon receiving the news that a friend or family member has cancer, especially if the person was not sick and was enthusiastically looking forward to future projects. As soon as we hear the word CANCER, we picture a shortened life. It is often subconscious, but this word has great power to kill due to this fearful reaction.

**Remember that many people do not die of cancer, but rather, because of their reaction to this illness and the numerous fears that this word CANCER provokes.**

What I suggest is taking some time after the initial shock, to verify what you are experiencing and what fears you are experiencing FOR YOURSELF in response to the announcement of your loved one's cancer. Take care to note them well, because I want to remind you that your ego makes you forget quickly the insights you have. Then give yourself the right to have these fears. It would be inhuman to try to make yourself believe you were not afraid. Allow yourself to really feel these fears in your body, to fill the places where they are located with white light.

It is also possible that if the person stricken with cancer is old and sick and no longer has a reason for living, you experience solace rather than fear upon hearing the news. In your view, it is this person's time to go, whether because of the cancer or another condition. This relief is often for one's own sake, if the person's condition demanded our time and energy to look after them. At the same time, we are happy to know that the person will finally stop suffering, merely existing on Earth, that they will finally be able to return to the world of the soul in order to join the rest of their family who is waiting for them.

Also take the time to experience that relief, it is not selfish, it is love for yourself and for the other person. You therefore must not feel guilty. Give yourself the right to be a person with limits. Feel that relief in your body and fill the space where it is located with white light.

## The fear of death

A major obstacle to dealing well with the news of a potentially life-threatening illness striking a friend or family member is the fear of death, which is very common among many people. I want to use this chapter to give a meaning to death that could be useful to you if you have this kind of fear.

WHAT IS DEATH? The dictionary tells us that death signifies the complete and definitive cessation of physical life. It represents the **natural cycle** of all life on the planet.

In humans, death is defined by the cessation of the functions of the physical body; medicine considers death as a failure; the relatives of the deceased consider it a tragedy, a misfortune, a disaster or even a calamity. The soul defines it as relief.

Actually, death is never an end, but always a continuation in another world. Rather than a door that closes, it is one that opens. Take the example of a tree that dies. The energy of the tree does not die. It continues to feed the ground: it becomes living soil. The one who understands that when apple blossoms fall, it is not a sad event but a sign that the tree is getting ready to produce apples, will also understand life and the principle of death.

It is impossible to destroy life and this is just as true for human life. The physical human body decays and feeds the earth while its soul returns to the world of the soul, its true home in the astral world, to prepare for new experiences. That is why we say the soul is immortal. Birth and death should therefore be considered as passages and not as a beginning and ending.

It remains nevertheless that it is human to experience sadness or fears when a loved one dies. The pain comes from the insecurity related to the unknown and the degree of attachment to that person. In those moments, it is legitimate to feel an emptiness, a sense of loss, powerlessness, anger, injustice or sometimes abandonment, related to that insecurity. We need to know, though, that no one owns anyone. Those who are inordinately affected by the death of a loved one must learn detachment.

For the deceased person, regardless of their age or the manner in which they died, their death signifies that they have completed their path in the context of this life. If it is not accepted by those close to them, it generally indicates that the deceased person has not accepted their own death.

Acceptance becomes absolutely necessary in order that everyone, the deceased as well as the living, may move on to new experiences. If you realize you have difficulty accepting the death of those dear to you or have a fear of death, you probably experience resistance to accepting changes in your life. When a person is liberated from their fear of death, they are also freed from many other fears.

Life consists of a continual resurrection. We are ceaselessly dying to one thing in order to be reborn to something else. Our cells constantly die and are reborn. To make it easier to accept death, you have only to speak to a person who has experienced clinical death for a few seconds or minutes. Most of these people state that they enter into a world of dazzling light filled with infinite love and that they feel very happy there. They no longer have a fear of dying after such an experience. It is reassuring to know that this represents a glorious moment for the soul as it returns home.

## Helping the person who has cancer

I know that we are generally inclined to want to help a loved one who is very sick and who, in our opinion, should not die now. But what is the best way to help them? Do you feel awkward in this kind of situation?

The first thing to do is ask the sick person if they need your help or support. If the answer is a firm *no*, do not insist, but tell them that if they change their mind, you are always available. Being so accustomed to experiencing things alone and convincing themselves that they are not suffering, it is very likely that this person wants to continue that way as they go about dealing with their situation.

That is why I suggest approaching them again later, but always with respect for their wishes. Above all, do not feel offended by their refusal. **They are not saying no to what you are, but only to the help you are offering them.** There is a strong possibility that the person will accept your help if they sense that your intention is helping them and not yourself and that you do not have any expectations of them. Too many people try to help others because they fear for themselves.

You might also offer to accompany them for their visits to the doctor, since they may be the type of person to want to ignore what they hear, for fear of facing reality. It is therefore a good idea for another person to go with them who can carefully note down the doctor's instructions.

When the person shows a desire for help, here are some suggestions you may want to use, only if you feel able to do so:

— Share what you felt when this cancer was announced, including the fear for yourself if they should die;

- Ask how they felt when this cancer was announced, what went through their head, their body, their soul, what fears they have for themselves if they were not able to continue the life they had before due to the effects of the cancer;

- Find out if they are comfortable with the idea of talking about the possibility of dying from this cancer.

If they agree, here are some suggestions of questions you might ask:

- *How do you feel at the thought of dying?*

- *Are you afraid for some of your loved ones? If you are, what in particular are you afraid of?*

- *How do you feel when you think of these fears?*

- *Are there people you will find particularly hard to leave? If so, why?*

- *Do you have any regrets about the way you have lived your life?*

- *Is there something you would really have liked to accomplish?*

- *Are you afraid you have missed an opportunity in a certain area?*

- *Are there certain people you would like to talk to before leaving this world?*

- *Do you believe in a life after death? Do you believe in God?*

- IF THEY SAY NO, you can then ask, *What do you think happens after we die?*

- *Where does that idea come from? Are you comfortable with that idea?*
- *Have you ever considered the possibility that there might be another way to understand death?*
- *Would you like to know more about the notions of life after death?*
- IF THEY SAY YES to the subject of life after death, *What do you think happens when you arrive in the world of the soul?*
- *Do you think God might be disappointed in you for something? If so, what would that be?*
- *Now, after looking from all angles at your possible death, let's talk about life. Do you want to live no matter what? If you do, why? In what way will it help you? What will it help you to be?*

It is important that you clearly respect the other person's answers, whatever they are, and especially not try to get them to change their mind. It's their body, their life, their decision to live or not. If they cannot or do not want to answer certain questions, you must above all not insist. The purpose of the questions is to help them reflect and find their own answers. It is not up to you to find an answer for the other person. Each question is a door that opens for them and only they can decide if they want to enter by that door or not. You must respect their limits.

Whatever you do, don't say things like, *Don't worry, you'll get through it.* So many people with cancer have confided to me that they are sick to death of hearing that stock phrase.

**It is much more important to encourage the person to talk about what they are experiencing than it is to tell them what we want for them.**

Another point to be attentive to is to avoid talking endlessly about their illness in their presence, because many people have had enough of talking only about that. It is important therefore to check if the person wants to talk before broaching the subject.

## Knowing ourselves by our reaction

What was your reaction to reading the preceding section? Did you think it would be impossible to be that direct with a person who has just learned they might die of cancer? Remember that those suggestions should be used ONLY if the person is open to receiving help.

I believe we should not wait until a person has died to start the process of mourning. How do we do that? By practising detachment. The greater your difficulty in facing the possibility of losing someone close to you, the more it means you are too attached to that person.

Detachment is done little by little, to the degree you become conscious that neither the person nor anything in this world belongs to you. That everything around you is transitory in your life and is there to answer a need. If you are the kind of person who can't throw out or give away anything in your house, the day will come when you feel completely overwhelmed by all those belongings. You will feel more and more suffocated and lacking in space. It's the same when we are unable to detach ourselves from people we love.

**Being detached does not mean abandoning or not loving.**

One can particularly like a piece of jewellery, for example, without being attached to it. The only way to become aware of your degree of attachment toward this item is if you end up losing it or having it stolen from you. Are you at peace living without it?

If not, you are still too attached to it. Your degree of attachment to objects is the same as it is to people. Why not start now to be more detached and to practise mourning?

You will know of course that the word *mourning* is also used figuratively: we mourn the loss of things. We say farewell to people but we speak of saying farewell to things too, when we mean that we accept being deprived of them for good, turning the page, moving on to something else. In other words, it's about realizing that it is time to become detached and move on and remember that life continues. If you have a hard time accepting the death of a dear one, it is because you are thinking of yourself and not of the other person who is following their life plan.

That's why it is so important that you practise acceptance. This will make it easier for you to adapt to each new phase of your life. Moreover, when you learn that one of your dear ones may possibly die of cancer or of any other illness, you will be in a much better position to help

If you are too attached, I would advise that you review the five normal stages of grief, so well explained by Elisabeth Kübler-Ross, psychiatrist, psychologist and pioneer of the "palliative care" approach for people at the end of life. Suppose you just learned that your spouse has cancer.

**The first stage is one of shock and denial**. When you first learn that someone close to you may die, you go into kind of a cocoon. You feel numbed and detached. You feel excluded from normal life and refuse to believe what's happening. *It can't be, it's not possible, they must have made a mistake and my sweetheart is going to come through this.*

**The second stage is anger**. *Why this damn sickness? It's not fair. Why is God doing this to us, when we have always been good people?* You are mad at the world, at life, at the circumstances, at the medical staff, you experience intense anger. You may even resent your loved one for being sick and possibly abandoning you. Guilt is often part of this stage.

**The third is bargaining**. During this stage, you think of everything that could still possibly be done to hold on to your dear one or return them to good health. You want your normal life back, your life "from before," you are prepared to change in order to achieve this. This is another form of denial. Even if you don't really believe in healing, you imagine that if you had acted differently in this or that situation, your sweetheart might not have this sickness.

Guilt also fuels this stage and you are filled with doubts and self-rejection. I know a woman who accused herself of having been a bad wife, of not having paid enough attention to her husband's diet and who said that it was therefore her fault that he had gotten colon cancer. During this stage, you may experience more physical problems, such as headaches, stomach aches, backaches, etc. The resistance felt at the idea of losing someone ends up sooner or later manifesting itself in the physical body. It is often at this time that people turn to prayer again and make promises to GOD.

**The fourth stage is depression, or bouts of depression, and grief.** Reality finally catches up with you at some point or other. You eventually realize that your life as a couple will never again be the same, whether your spouse dies or not. This illness is a turning point in your life and you experience disillusionment. You understand that the dreams and plans you had with this person may never be realized. You are overwhelmed by a sadness that may even give way to depression.

This stage may also involve resignation if you have no more resistance in you. At that point, when your three bodies – mental, emotional and physical – are no longer able to resist, illness may result.

**Let us move into the fifth and final stage, acceptance.** This is the most important stage. So that your grieving process may finally be concluded, you must welcome acceptance. Given that the goal of this book is to help you accept yourself and all the decisions that others make, why not practise now? Then, you will not have to go through all those painful stages. It would be ideal to be able to move immediately into acceptance, but this is only possible if you have already learned detachment in other situations of grief or loss.

I would remind you that accepting does not mean conceding or agreeing. To accept is to respect what is happening, it is to observe, it is to know that whatever may happen, there is always a good reason, and there is always something useful you can learn from it.

You know that your grieving process has concluded with acceptance when:

— You gradually become accustomed to your new reality;

— You gradually open yourself to new projects and dreams.

— You think of your former relationship, but not constantly, and without such intense pain.

However, each person's grief is unique. Certain stages can take longer or be experienced more deeply than others. Moreover, these stages do not necessarily happen in precise chronological order. You can feel anger one day, great sadness the next, then anger again or guilt the following day.

The stages of grief are lived differently depending on the wounds that are activated in you when you receive the news of the cancer or the death of your loved one. If you are capable of doing your own grieving well, you will be in a much better position to help another person go through each of these stages

Discovering what you need to learn through the illness, and possibly the death, of the other person is of great use to you and can greatly facilitate your acceptance of the situation. *How could the illness or death of another person whom I love so much be of any use to me?* you will say. This experience helps you become conscious of the degree of attachment or possession you have in your life. It helps you become conscious of your capacity for letting go, for not wanting to control everything in your life or in the life of another. It helps you to become conscious of what is directing your life: your ego or your heart.

Resistance always comes from the ego. When you are in your heart, it is easier for you to accept the decision of another soul, its life path, even if you do not understand why a person would choose that type of illness to learn something that is important to them.

**We never need to understand the decisions others make, only to accept them.**

Many people never conclude their grieving process, feeling such a strong attachment to those they love. I have often met parents who still mourn the death of their child after more than twenty years. I know they blame themselves, aways thinking about what they should have said or done differently.

Others experience this in regard to their parents with whom they may have had many conflicts, telling themselves they should have reconciled with them sooner and that now it is too late. These are typical examples of people who do not accept themselves.

The sickness and death of a loved one should on the contrary have served them as a means of becoming conscious of this non-acceptance. Some will choose perhaps subconsciously to attract a cancer or another illness in turn, precisely in order to become conscious of it, if they do not wish to acknowledge it now. Either way, there is always an important lesson to be learned for anyone dealing with this same situation.

You will find concrete methods to help you learn greater self-acceptance in the next chapter.

# Chapter Nine

## Discovering the power of love

This last chapter is dedicated to offering you as many ways as possible to love yourself instead of rejecting yourself, in order to help you:

- become aware once again of the extraordinary person you are;
- expand your limits by ceasing to believe in powerlessness;
- reconnect with your divine power which can heal and prevent cancer.

I want to clarify that this chapter is addressed to anyone whose intention it is to learn to love themselves more. On the other hand, my writing is addressed particularly to people who have suffered or are still suffering from cancer. If, however, you are reading this book for information purposes only, that can be an excellent means of preventing cancer.

What does loving yourself really mean? If you are among those who have read several of my books and participated in numerous workshops, you have surely heard what follows here countless times. Nevertheless, I want to remind you that our ego plays such tricks on us that at times we believe we will always remember everything we have learned.

Unfortunately, this is rarely true, especially with respect to newly acquired knowledge in the spiritual domain, which needs to be put into practice in order to have any effect and to be truly integrated in a permanent way. For example, the stages of reconciliation and forgiveness are often forgotten even by people who have been hearing about them for years.

Recently, a friend of longstanding, who had completed the entire *Listen to Your Body* training program several years ago, confided to me in an e-mail a painful event that she experienced with a member of her family, another woman with whom she had always been on good terms. She wrote, *I never want to see her or hear about her again. Her words and actions are so unfair that I no longer wish to suffer the pain of being in contact with her.*

I was immediately able to sense that her suffering – the rejection experienced from this woman – was so strong that she completely forgot everything she had learned. When I reminded her that she wouldn't stop suffering until she applied what she had learned, that is, until she remembered that everything she attracts is hers and is only a reflection of what is going on inside her, she did not resist. She knew very well that it was true, even if she could not apply it right away. She was even surprised to note that what she had put into practice many times before in her life had suddenly disappeared from her memory at the time when this situation occurred, because her pain was too great.

It is important to distinguish between experience, and knowledge. Knowledge refers to learning something new while experience involves putting it into practice, and thus acquiring a new consciousness of what we have learned through practice.

Some people believe they have deep consciousness because they have read a lot or participated in all sorts of workshops.

But it is only knowledge that they have acquired. They are the first to insist they are right in discussions, believing they know it all. This type of attitude is called *intellectual pride*.

**In reality, true consciousness comes only with experience.**

The same is true of forgiveness. Reading about the stages or hearing about them in a workshop has little to do with the reality of experiencing it. It is only after going through this type of experience several times that you can truly be conscious of all the benefits it can bring you. This is why it is important to start off by practising with the less painful wounds in order to finally be reconciled with others and forgive yourself in the most difficult situations.

## True love

Here are some of the characteristics of self-love that we have been teaching at the *Listen to Your Body* school for over thirty years:

- Respect yourself;
- Give yourself the right to be human;
- Lead your life by listening to your own needs;
- Make requests and be willing to receive from others;
- Make commitments before having expectations;
- Remember that you are the only one responsible for yourself;

– Accept, observe and welcome, even if your ego does not agree.

I will now expand on each of these notions, in order to assist you better with healing the wounds of rejection and injustice which are at the root of all cancers.

## Respect yourself

To respect yourself means to recognize that you need space in order to live, just like everything else that lives on Earth, the plants and animals and all of nature. This vital space is needed for your mental, emotional and physical bodies.

**Mental**: your thoughts, ideas and knowledge belong to you and you do not need to change them to feel loved by someone else. Taking your space means daring to state your ideas or your opinion and especially accepting that if others do not agree with what you say, they are not thereby rejecting you, but simply do not have the same opinion as you, since their knowledge and experiences differ from yours.

**Emotional**: Your desires, feelings and goals belong to you and even if they don't suit your friends and family, you don't have to change them in order to feel loved. You have the right to have goals that are different, just as they do. And especially, have enough self-esteem to dare to go toward the goals you have set for yourself.

**Physical**: Your physical space includes all your assets, your possessions, your money and your time and you can use these as you see fit. You can therefore decide what you want in your life, because you will always be the only person who can assume the consequences of your decisions.

If someone else tries to make you believe that what you possess, what you do or what you are, bothers them and they feel constrained to assume the consequences of your choices, it is simply an indication that this person does not know how to respect their own space. THEY ARE NOT TELLING YOU THAT YOU ARE OF NO VALUE AND THEY ARE NOT REJECTING YOU. Their problem comes from their own interpretation or their beliefs regarding your attitude. This person does not realize that by trying to penetrate into your space, they lose their own. They are also a reflection of you.

If you do not respect yourself in what you are, what you do and what you have, it is certain that those around you cannot do it for you. We cannot reap from others what we have not sown. You should use the people around you to become conscious of how much you do or do not respect yourself, which will help you to orient yourself toward greater love for yourself.

**Those around you are but a reflection of your attitude toward yourself.**

In a parallel way, ask the people around you if they feel that you often infringe on their physical, emotional or mental space. That will help you to understand that if you do not respect them in their space, it is a sign that you do not respect yourself. I want to come back to the example of the agent at the airport who was insulted that I did not stop to have my passport and boarding pass checked. I am certain that this woman felt that I did not respect her just as I felt she did not respect me, by the way she shouted at me in a loud voice in front of several people.

## Give yourself the right to be human

It has been stated many times over in this book that if you have attracted cancer into your life, it was caused by your wounds of rejection and injustice, the latter appearing especially to help you not feel the rejection. These are the two wounds that push you to live according to some unattainable goal. In fact, you have to admit that you must have been very demanding of yourself all through your life, to the point of becoming eternally dissatisfied.

**The person toward whom you are the most unfair is yourself, with the result that you feel even more rejected.**

All that to say you were unable to give yourself the right to be human with faults, limits, fears, weaknesses or unhealed wounds. You surely criticized yourself a great deal for all kinds of things. When someone criticized you, it only confirmed what you already believed about yourself. Since this non-acceptance is often unconscious, you may still be experiencing great anger when others criticize you, not wishing to face that you are criticizing yourself to the same degree. However this anger is very well repressed, except during those moments when you reach your limits and your wound of injustice then gets the upper hand. This wound then pushes you to resist and you openly blame the other person who is criticizing you.

When it is your wound of rejection that is operating, you say nothing, you withdraw or you leave. When you protest openly, it is rather your wound of injustice that is taking over. Your wound of rejection causes you furthermore to criticize yourself for having needs, desires or beliefs with which others disagree, and this makes you feel guilty.

Start right now to accept the fact that every person on this planet is human, with highs and lows, strengths and weaknesses, etc. Know that the ideal of perfection that you have created for yourself is not realistic.

**True divine perfection is manifested when you give yourself the right to be human without any criticism or value judgment.**

To know to what degree you give yourself permission to be human, check again with the people around you how much you want to change them by criticizing them or judging them. I would remind you that every aspect of another person that you judge, you judge in yourself as well, even if you are not conscious of it and thinking you never behave that way, especially when you force yourself to be the opposite. All your soul desires is for you to claim your right to be what you are, all of the time. It knows that you will then gradually succeed in being more of what you want to be.

This acceptance is the only answer to several of the questions posed in Chapter One. Let's take, *Why do some heavy smokers never get cancer while tobacco is considered the leading cause of lung cancer?* I have heard of many people who smoked all their life and yet, according to the autopsy done after their death, had the pink lungs of a non-smoker. Why? Because they gave themselves permission to have this kind of desire. They smoked because they enjoyed it, fully savouring every cigarette WITHOUT FEELING GUILTY. That is how we know we are acting out of love: there is no judgment or accusation of any kind whatsoever on our part or on the part of others.

I am not saying everyone should smoke: it is obvious that the body must use its energy to flush out anything it does not need in the cigarette and that this energy could be used for something more constructive. But I've never met anyone who doesn't have desires that may require extra work and effort from the physical body.

There are people who convince themselves that they are listening to the needs of their physical body, but they are doing it out of fear by constantly monitoring and controlling themselves. This attitude is the very opposite of acceptance and they often find themselves losing control in some other area of their life. Finally, they attract what they are afraid of, as I explained above.

What will your decision be? To accept yourself as a human being with your strengths and weaknesses so you will succeed in loving yourself and improving your quality of life? Or to have unrealistic expectations of yourself and live in fear?

## The listen-to-your-body triangle

I want to come back to certain things I have already said in this book, because the lessons that follow from the great spiritual law of life bear frequent repeating.

**The way you are with yourself is the way you are with others and the way others are with you.**

What is even more interesting is that what happens between another person and you is always of equal intensity for each of you. The fears and emotions experienced are as strong for the other person as they are for you.

Have you ever been in a difficult situation with another person and thought that you were suffering much more than they were? It may have seemed that way but that is not the case.

This happens because each of us has different levels of consciousness, just as we show what we are experiencing in varying degrees. Take the very rigid person who appears indifferent in the face of misfortune. It does not mean that they do not experience great inner distress, but rather that they repress or deny it by controlling themselves.

Recalling this triangle will make it easier to have compassion for others and for yourself, which is an important criterion of whether you love yourself. Since you have the power to create your life yourself, why not use this triangle to bring about the realization of your desires? For instance, if you are seeking to be surrounded by supportive people rather than critical people, this spiritual law of life tells you that all you have to do is be supportive toward yourself and others and people will be that way with you. It becomes a virtuous circle rather than a vicious one provoked by criticism.

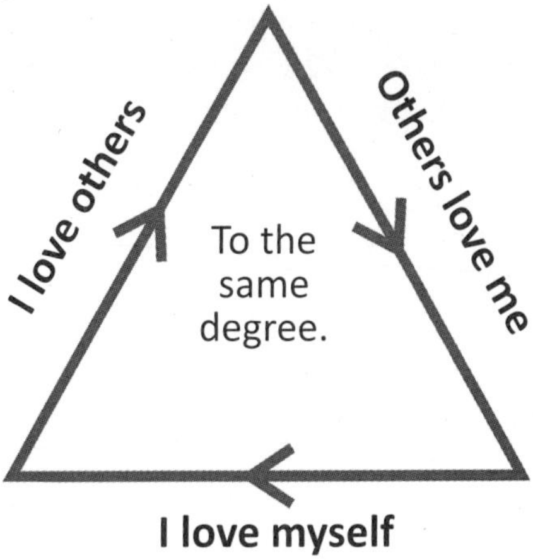


## Lead your life by listening to your own needs

In Chapter Seven, I stated the importance of taking the decision to live for yourself. But do you really know what you want, what you need? Are you the kind of person who checks to see if what you want is bothering others or if they agree? Are you inclined to check with your friends and family how they feel about the fact that you are taking care to listen to your needs? Surely you observed in the examples of cancer cited in Chapter Five that already early on in childhood, these people did not have the right to listen to their own needs. Denise expressed it very well when she said she *was allowed only desires that were pleasing to her mother*.

When we were young, very few of us learned that we had the right to have desires and needs, especially if our parents didn't agree with them. It is therefore a learning process that each of us needs to decide to undertake at some point or other during our life. So, why not right now?

If you have a hard time figuring out what you need, ask yourself the following question: *If all the circumstances were perfect right now and it didn't upset anyone, what would I want for myself?* When you have the answer, make sure you also know what this desire, once manifested, would help you to BE.

Let's take the example of Julie who developed thyroid cancer. If she had asked herself this question, she would surely have received the following answer: *I want to stop working and stay at home with my children*. This reply in itself represents a desire. Everything to do with *having* and *doing* is considered a desire. As for the real need, it has to do with *being*. People with the wound of rejection who do not give themselves the right to be or to exist have an even greater need to ask themselves the following question: *When this desire is realized, what will it help me to BE?* In Julie's case, the answer would have been: *to be independent, to be free to decide for myself*. She has just become aware of a part of her life path: she needs to experience being independent, being free to decide, without feeling guilty.

Can you see that with this kind of exercise, it becomes easier to grant yourself the right, or give yourself permission, to use various ways (like realizing your desires) of gradually becoming what you need to be in order to experience true happiness?

Be aware that it is impossible for anyone to have desires that will get the approval of all their loved ones. To look for that will only bring frustration and finally create a feeling of powerlessness. It is one impossibility, among so many, which countless people unfortunately continue to believe in. In contrast, it is quite possible for you to realize desires that make you go WOW. Consequently it is very important that you distinguish between a possibility, an impossibility and powerlessness.

**Possibility and impossibility derive from reality, while powerlessness derives from a reaction on the part of your ego to a situation or a person.**

In summary, you must once and for all adjust to the idea that you are entitled to have needs that are different from other people's needs. It is even essential to allow yourself to have them. Remember also that when you feel powerless, it is not your fears that make you powerless, but **the fact that you believe you are powerless that creates your fears.**

The more you authorize yourself to listen to your own needs, the easier it will be to accept that others have desires and needs different from yours. To know whether you have that acceptance, check your reaction when a friend or family member informs you of a desire with which you do not agree. Do you try to make them change their mind or even categorically forbid them to go ahead? Or might you on the other hand be prepared to help them despite disagreeing with their desire – just for the pleasure of doing them a favour? I suggest checking with people you are close to as to how they see you in this regard.

Do you stop living because the life choices of your family members and friends don't suit you or upset you? For example, I know several grandmothers who are unhappy because they disagree with the way their children are raising their grandchildren. They are convinced that if their son or daughter and their spouse listened to their advice, everyone would be much better off. They can get so worked up about it that they may end up with uterine cancer, a type of cancer that represents the family nest.

Others believe it is their fault if family members aren't getting along and are experiencing difficulties. No, each and every one of us has a different life path and obviously you cannot control everything, just as others cannot control you. This attitude would be the opposite of genuine love for yourself and for others.

It would be wise to remember that your environment is your own responsibility. If someone or something is harming you or bothering you and you allow this to prevent you from listening to your needs, it is up to you to change either your environment or your way of thinking. Consequently you must choose and decide something else.

On the other hand, do not forget that whatever your desire or your need, nothing will manifest in your life as long as you do not take action. The fact of facing what you really want is an excellent way to change the image of yourself that you have created. When you do this, you will realize that you are no longer alone, that the Universe is always at work helping those who take a decision to help themselves. You have surely heard the saying, *Heaven helps those who help themselves.*

## Make requests and be willing to receive from others

In order for any desire to manifest, it is very possible that you will have to make requests, but that you will not dare to do so for fear of being refused. When someone says *no* to one of your requests, he or she is not saying no to what you ARE but to what you are requesting. By keeping everything inside like that, and not knowing what you want, others are unable to offer you anything. You then get confirmation once more that they do not love you – in your eyes – and you thus continue to feel rejected. What a vicious circle, wouldn't you say?

Can you see just how much your ego is playing tricks on you when you are not yourself and you let yourself be convinced that no one loves you? It is your ego, with that fear of not being good enough, making you believe you are too insignificant to be truly loved

How do you react when someone offers to help you when you did not ask them for help? It is quite likely that your initial reaction is to refuse and say that you can manage just fine on your own. Why is that? Because you do not feel worthy of receiving help, especially if you consider you do not deserve it. Do you realize that when you refuse like that, the other person may also feel rejected by you? Was it your intention to reject them? Certainly not. Your refusal was no doubt motivated by your belief that you do not deserve to receive help from someone to whom you have never given anything.

It is time you became more aware of this type of situation, remembering that the intentions of others may also be different than you think. It is your wound of rejection that is distorting everything; it can easily make you believe that others are rejecting you when that is totally false. You can see that in this type of situation the two wounds of rejection and injustice are very often activated.

I suggest you try the following experiment: quite simply say, *thank you so much, that's very kind*, when someone offers you help or advice, at the same time sensing the pleasure the other person will gain from helping you. If it is advice, welcome it, knowing that the other person's intent is to help. Afterwards, you will do with their advice as you wish.

I don't know how many times I have approached a person suffering from rejection with the words, *May I suggest something that I sincerely believe can help you achieve this task more easily?* only to have them refuse my offer. In their wound of rejection, the person does not dare say anything, but I can tell immediately, from their withdrawn and tight-lipped manner, that they are listening to me politely without really hearing what I am saying. Because of their suffering, they think something like *That's it, she is is telling me I'm not doing my work properly, that I'm no good at it and should be more like her. She's never satisfied*. When it is the wound of injustice that is activated, people are more able to speak up. When it is the wound of rejection, they keep their feelings to themselves and repress them.

If only you took the time to pay yourself compliments every day, and became conscious of just how special, gifted, talented, hard-working and dedicated you are, you would know then that you have the right to make requests of others and get help from them. You can dare to allow yourself to receive from others even when you have not made a request or even if you have never yet given anything to that person.

**By refusing help, you are fighting against divine justice, which always wishes that you should reap what you sow.**

Are you aware of the numerous times that you helped other people? I admit that your motivation may have been that you wanted to feel loved by that person, but why would you not accept this help from others who assuredly have the same motivation you did? You are not the only one who has so much difficulty loving yourself that you have to look for this love outside yourself. The law of reciprocity stipulates clearly that you do not necessarily receive from the person to whom you have given. You may have done a favour sometime for someone in a store and then find that a favour is returned to you by one of your neighbours.

Every person aspires to receive and give in love, that is to say, without any specific expectations being attached by the giver. They are two sides of the same thing. When you give only for the pleasure of it, you are generally inclined to verify with the other person whether they want your help. If the person refuses and you wanted to give out of love, it will be easier for you to accept their refusal, knowing they are just expressing their need and not rejecting you. It is also possible that the other person still has a lot of difficulty to accept being at the receiving end.

When you know how to give out of love, you receive out of love. Consequently, you will be able to connect with the pleasure the other person experiences when they help you or give you something. On the other hand, very few people are able today to give and receive out of love, most of them doing it much more in order to be loved. It is therefore preferable not to judge yourself if you still find it hard to always receive and give out of love. You have only to remind yourself in that case, that it is your wounds that are operating and make you react that way.

When someone refuses your help and you immediately feel rejected, to the point of blaming yourself for being useless and unimportant and believing that that is why the other person acted that way, ask yourself the following question: *Did I want to help the other person in order to feel loved or simply to make them happy?* This has proven to be an excellent way of becoming aware yet again of how much and how frequently our wound of rejection is activated. Not just when you are afraid others will reject you, but also when you reject yourself and when you are afraid that others feel rejected by you.

In conclusion, when another person refuses your help, they are not rejecting YOU, they are only expressing THEIR need at that moment, which has nothing to do with what you are. When you in turn refuse help from someone else, you are acting in the same way and there is therefore no form of rejection. When you live consciously and accept this fact, the way you say *no* will be different and it will not be in any way reactive.

## Make commitments before you have expectations

If you find it hard to receive, it is very likely that you often have expectations of others. Since you often keep them to yourself, or you don't express them clearly, this causes you a lot of frustration, and ultimately to feel a sense of powerlessness.

No one is entitled to have expectations without an agreement having been established first. This ability to have clear and precise agreements is very difficult for the person suffering from rejection, given the difficulty they have communicating and how hard they find it to be truly conscious of their needs. We have moreover seen this among the cancer cases described in Chapter Five. By refusing to feel and making themselves believe that everything is going fine, it is very easy to ignore what we want in life, especially the help that would be particularly useful to us.

As you become more conscious of the importance of this wound in your life, you will more quickly sense the frustration or disappointment that you experience in various situations and with certain people. As soon as you perceive this feeling, take a few moments to ask yourself what your expectations were at that exact moment. You will realize almost right away that there was no prior established agreement. Remember that it takes two to make an agreement.

Another important point to remember is that no one can commit to BEING anything. Consequently, we cannot require of anyone that they promise us to BE something.

**Commitments and agreements can only be made with regard to *doing* and *having*. They cannot be made with regard to *being*.**

Let's go back to the case of Denise, whose mother refused to let her children call her Mom. There was never any agreement made between her and her mother that she should be called anything else. The same thing happened with her husband. He had never promised that he would abstain from any addictions when they married. When we make a request with expectations, that doesn't make it an agreement. In fact, it looks more like an order and we expect the other person to obey. We think (wrongly) that if the other person obeys us, without there having been a true agreement, it is proof of their love.

We can even make ourselves believe that there is an agreement while the other person has never said yes, but has only heard the request. Here is an example from my first marriage: The week before my birthday, I said to my then husband one day, *You know, dear, it's my birthday next week and I'm reminding you that my favourite restaurant is the one in the Queen Elizabeth Hotel.* He gave me a little smile without saying a word. I was convinced that he had just made a commitment even though he was only half-listening. I had the habit of often speaking to him while he was busy with something else, and I would assume he had really heard me. The following week, he completely forgot my birthday.

As you can imagine, he never did promise when we married that he would remember my birthday every year and, what's more, to celebrate it at my favourite restaurant. You can guess the rest. I was unhappy, angry and frustrated, told myself I would pay him back when it was his birthday. There you have one reason, among others, why our marriage ended after fifteen years. We had never learned to make clear and specific agreements. I constantly looked for proof that he loved me because I didn't love myself enough.

How can the other person feel like offering us proof of their love when our demands on them go completely against the laws of unconditional love? It's like wanting to harvest carrots when you have planted radishes. The law that says that we always reap what we sow applies in every field – physical as well as psychological.

If you recognize yourself in these descriptions, you can see that you are someone who often has expectations without an agreement between you and the other party. It indicates you are doing the same thing with yourself: you have many expectations of yourself but did not make a real commitment.

I have given an example of commitment in the realm of doing. Now, let us see how that is different from the realm of being. Suppose that you are often inclined to escape into your thoughts when you find yourself in the presence of someone who intimidates you. Since it is impossible to make a commitment on the level of BEING, you cannot promise yourself you will always be attentive at every instant. You can on the other hand promise yourself – take the decision – to take three deep breaths when you feel you are about to withdraw into your thoughts. After that, you are perhaps going to realize that this promise is beyond your limits and you are unable to keep it. Instead of judging yourself and feeling guilty, welcome yourself with your limits and make yourself a different promise that is less demanding. You could promise yourself, for example, that you are going to do it every other time.

I have indicated repeatedly in this book just how difficult it is for people with the wounds of rejection and injustice to respect their limits and how demanding they are of themselves. This is why I emphasize the point that you should treat yourself more kindly, be less demanding of yourself and make sure that the commitments you make to yourself are realistic before you have so many expectations.

## Remember that you are the only one responsible for yourself

This notion of responsibility is indispensable if we are to succeed in healing all our wounds, both spiritual and physical. This great lack of love for ourselves is due to the fact that we forget that we are constantly responsible for our life and therefore the only creator of all that happens to us.

In everything I have been able to learn in my life and in what I have been teaching for over thirty years, this notion of responsibility is the one that brings the most resistance from the ego. The ego always wants in fact to make us believe that when we encounter any problem whatsoever, it is another person that is causing it. It is convinced that everything that happens to us comes from without and not from within.

In order to learn to truly love and truly forgive, to be able to apply the notion of the mirror, accept the notion of the triangle and stop having expectations, we need first of all to accept and practise the notion of responsibility, as explained in Chapter Six.

If you feel incapable of this, then what is written in this book will have hardly any effect on you because of your resistance. I know that when faced with certain situations, like the real-life experiences described in Chapter Five, it is normal and human to believe that we never intended for these things to happen to us and never intended for our parents to have such attitudes toward us. Another belief of the ego.

Another example comes to mind. Francine healed herself from a massive carcinoma, a cellular mass in her shoulder. Francine was the fifth child and her birth had not in the least been anticipated, any more than it had been desired. Her mother used to call her *the accident* until she was fourteen, but one day she rebelled and told her mother not to call her that anymore.

You may be thinking, *It was normal that poor Francine felt rejected, after being called* the *"accident" by her whole family. Never having asked for that, it was obviously not her fault. Indeed, she would surely have preferred to be welcomed from the time she was born. Really, wasn't it her family's fault if Francine thought of herself as worthless and stupid and felt she wasn't even entitled to a first name?*

That is very much the ego's reaction. For the ego, it is impossible to understand and accept that we are all creator-gods and are constantly creating our life, whether pleasant or unpleasant. It cannot accept that we have this great power to choose nor can it admit that when we choose to make something happen that we do not want, it is truly the result of a decision on our part, whether it was a conscious decision or not. It always tries to make us believe that if things aren't going well in our life, it is someone else's fault or due to some external factor.

**And how about you? What do you choose with your thoughts, beliefs and actions?**

**To make things happen that you do want or that you don't want?**

In Francine's case, why did she attract birth into a family where she felt so rejected? Quite simply, in order to meet the needs of her soul. Initially decided in the world of the soul before we are born, our life path is determined by the needs of our soul and not by our desires.

**In life, what happens to us is always a response to our NEEDS and not to our DESIRES.**

Our needs are a function of our being and are therefore spiritual in nature, while a desire originates in the material realm, seeking to provide what we would like physically, emotionally and mentally. As most of us are not conscious enough to know what our soul needs in order to live in true love, our inner GOD draws us like a magnet toward the family and environment we need in order to manifest our life path, in each of our lives.

One might say, then, that Francine was attracted by this type of family because she needed above all to work on her wound of rejection in her present life. She must learn to truly love herself rather than reject herself. As we always reap what we sow, reaping such rejection was triggered by the rejection she had felt for such a long time toward herself and toward others. From when she was young, Francine felt a great deal of rejection from her mother and her older sister, as well as from her classmates who made fun of her when she attended a convent school because she was a farmer's daughter.

These people from whom she suffered so much rejection most certainly suffered the same thing from Francine. Remember that any feeling of rejection – as well as any emotion – experienced in a relationship is always felt by both parties with equal intensity. Everything depends on the degree of consciousness and how deeply we feel.

What happened to that entire family was what they needed. If on the other hand you asked each of them if they wanted to experience that kind of rejection in the family, you can imagine that none of them would have said yes. Let's remember that our desires come from the emotional and mental bodies and that these are unaware of the true needs of the soul.

Our needs emerge directly from our inner GOD, an omniscient GOD that knows everything about us since the creation of our soul. Our inner GOD knows all that we need in order to return to the light, which all earthly souls aspire to. That sublime moment will only be possible the moment we give ourselves the right to be human, with our imperfections and our wounds, as I have already explained.

It is imperative, then, to be more conscious of the fact that you are constantly creating your life based on your choices of actions, reactions and decisions. If your life is not functioning as you would like, in happiness and inner peace, you automatically know that you are not listening to your soul's greatest need, the need to love yourself.

Moreover, if you do not accept that it is always you who attract all the situations and people you need, you will be inclined to blame others for your misfortunes. You will think furthermore that if others are responsible for your happiness, you are responsible for theirs. That will make you a controlling person in your behaviour toward others. All the time you spend concerned for the happiness of others will be time wasted for you. Have you not understood yet that you are on this Earth only for yourself? For the healing of your wounds? To help guide your soul back to the light? No one else can do this for you, and you cannot do it for anyone else. It is your ego that makes you believe otherwise. You have a choice whether to let it direct your life or not.

The most harmful consequence of not adhering to the notion of responsibility is the sense of guilt you experience as well as the guilt you lay on others, as explained earlier in this book.

## Accept and observe, even if your ego doesn't agree

I will conclude this explanation of the magnificent notions of true love with the one I consider exceptionally important, that is, understanding what is meant by the word *ACCEPT*. I therefore repeat here what has already been written in Chapter Six concerning reconciliation and forgiveness.

**To accept does not mean to agree. It means to recognize, welcome and observe a fact or a person. That is to say, there is no judgment of anything or anyone being either good or bad.**

If it is hard for you to accept yourself, it is because you think you ARE what you DO or what you POSSESS. **You are much more than that.** Accepting yourself is the only way to become again what you want to be.

This means that every time you notice you feel rejected or realize you are rejecting another person, you need to accept and observe that this wound is still present in you. Accept the fact that you could not help but allow it to influence you regarding the situation rather than judging yourself, blaming yourself and especially trying to ignore everything in order not to feel your wound.

**To accept is to authorize yourself to be what you do not want to be, while at the same time remembering what you want to be.**

With this type of acceptance, I can assure you that one day, you will reach the point where you are more often what you want to be and still give yourself permission to be human with weaknesses and limits.

To heal your wound of rejection, be more alert to situations that make you want to withdraw, escape or hold yourself back from saying what you think and what you really feel. By doing this, you will become aware that your fear of being rejected has just gotten the better of you. Look at this fear, welcome it by getting in touch with the little child in you that is afraid. You are not being bad when you are afraid. You are just being human.

## Love yourself physically

The more you accept yourself as you are each day, the more you will authorize yourself to love your physical self. It will not be easy at first, because the greater the wound of rejection, the more people deprive themselves of all physical pleasure.

Since the three material dimensions of the human cannot be dissociated, when there is a transformation on either the physical, emotional or mental level, it is felt on the other two levels and immediately has an influence on them. In other words, the three levels are constantly affecting one another.

You are without a doubt aware that for several years now, we have all been subjected to increasing amounts of pollution – air pollution, noise, toxic food and drink, electromagnetic waves – which has an effect on our energy and causes us more and more stress. All of us have to continually make our immune system work harder in order to counteract the effects of these toxic substances. It is therefore more urgent than ever that each of us do everything in our power to help ourselves, which means taking decisions consistent with a love of self.

I would remind you that the natural order of things is for your three bodies to be at the service of your soul, that is, the material at the service of the spiritual. In this book, I have especially insisted on the spiritual aspect and thus on true love, the acceptance of our entire being, whether expressed in positive or negative behaviours. The suggestions described below are meant to assist you on the physical and psychological level; they can only help you get onto the path of taking charge of your life rather than letting yourself to be controlled by external factors.

To begin with, here are several methods that will help you on the physical level; they will be all the more effective if you take the time to feel the pleasure experienced by your body.

*Pay attention to what you eat*

Take the trouble to try new foods and thus discover new sensations. Many experts, like Dr. Richard Béliveau, have done a great deal of research and written excellent books on the subject. Even if you only make small changes in the beginning, if you do it with the intention of helping your body as much as possible, you can be certain your body will feel it, and that it will be beneficial for you.

On the other hand, I invite you to use your discernment well, for there are many schools of thought on the subject of food recommended to people with cancer. For example, Chinese medicine suggests eating meat, especially pork. Indian medicine (Ayurveda) suggests a vegetarian diet accompanied by dairy products and sugar in order to have a balanced diet. Finally, Western naturopathic medicine advises against sugar and dairy.

The most important thing here is that everything you ingest should basically be eaten with love for yourself and not out of fear. Otherwise, you will become rigid about your way of eating and that will not help you in the least toward the path of healing. On the contrary, it will only make you feel guilty if you deviate from what you think is best for you.

**To know if it is out of love for yourself, ask yourself if you would continue to eat this way if your cancer were to disappear.**

Whatever you decide to take – food, drink or medication – your primary intention should always be to help yourself regain your natural energy, that is, an energy that flows freely and isn't blocked. If instead it is out of fear of suffering, sickness or death, you will lose rather than gain energy. This is true for any kind of help. If, for example, you only see an osteopath so he can take away your pain, there will be no end to the treatment. If instead you seek to reconnect with your natural energy, this therapist's assistance will have a very different effect on you. **Everything depends on YOUR intention and not on the intention of the person helping you.** Only YOU have the power to make a difference in your life.

*Take the time to really taste your food*

By eating slowly and allowing yourself to savour, you will taste life more fully. You will feel more like offering yourself physical pleasure, something that is often difficult for people who suffer from rejection. Moreover, this can only improve your sexual life. In fact, there is a direct connection between sexual enjoyment and your ability to taste and to feel pleasure while eating and drinking.

*Start your day with physical exercises*

Be sure to include, as one of the stretch exercises you choose, one where you pull your arms back, as this helps open up the thorax. The thorax is generally inclined to contract due to the wound of rejection. Studies done by the World Fund For Cancer Research have also shown that physical activity is associated with a significantly reduced risk of getting certain types of cancer. You will certainly be aware of all the benefits of physical exercise, mainly the prevention of cardio-vascular illnesses, so why not go for it? What a nice way to demonstrate to yourself that you know you deserve to be loved!

*Breathe clean air everyday*

Chinese medicine holds that all cancers are related to the lungs and the skin (the two organs that breathe), cancer being caused when these organs are unable to take in sufficient air. Many acupuncturists treat blockages of this type in people with cancer. We know very well that air is what every living thing on Earth needs most. With the first inhalation, life begins and with the last exhalation, it ends. The lungs are therefore a symbol of life and of death. You can see why it is very important to make a habit of breathing properly.

When you breathe in, take the time to feel the air filling your lungs and your rib cage expanding. Even if you only take five minutes in the morning and five in the evening to practise deep breathing, preferably outdoors, your body will feel all the better for it.

Breathing in a more balanced way helps you to be calmer mentally, allowing you to hear the little voice of your heart speaking. It has also been shown that proper breathing promotes better circulation, thus helping the blood flow to all the organs.

Have you ever had the experience of going to an appointment for some kind of professional care – from a doctor, a therapist, a masseuse or an esthetician, for example, and the person providing the care arrives all out of breath and scrambling to get organized while at the same time they start to talk to you and work on you? It has happened to me a few times and I immediately knew I would never come back for this person's services again. How can they give their client their full attention when they are in that kind of state? And furthermore, they are subjecting their client to the stress they have brought with them into their office or clinic.

If this person thought of taking the time, even just a few minutes, to breathe deeply, their quality of care would be so much improved. Moreover, it is certain that this kind of person is not thinking about encouraging their client to breathe properly. I often reflect that if all therapists could regularly remind their clients to take a few deep breaths during a session, treatment results would surely be greatly enhanced.

This reminds me of the stress I feel whenever I have a dental appointment for cleaning. I have barely arrived and I already look forward to leaving. In fact, just the deep breaths I take during the work is all I need to help me not be tense about the treatment. Although the hygienist and dentist are kind and efficient, neither of them thinks of telling me to breathe.

To summarize, a few minutes of silent, conscious, deep breathing several times a day will benefit you greatly. I know that with the increasingly hectic lives we lead, it is especially difficult to grant ourselves quiet time alone. On the other hand, it is precisely because of this frantic pace that we need it more than ever.

**If you cannot be alone with yourself, how can you expect others to want to be with you?**

Heart-focused breathing, which is becoming increasingly popular, is another breathing method that I frequently practise myself. It owes its popularity to the U.S.-based Institute of HeartMath, where several doctors and scientists have made amazing discoveries such as the fact that this type of breathing helps alter DNA.

Here is a summary of their recommendations: To release yourself from being dominated by mental considerations or certain emotions, shift your attention to the region of the heart. Imagine that you are inhaling and exhaling through the heart to help you keep your attention focused there. Breathe this way at least ten times while saying to yourself silently, *I breathe in – pause – I breathe out – pause*. This practice will promote being in harmony with your heart.

*Walk*

Breathing well will be much more effective if you take a walk at the same time, a walk in nature if possible, or even better, in the mountains. Have you ever heard that in our cities, the atmosphere is now called the *technosphere*? We are bombarded my multiple waves emanating from radio and television signals, from Wi-fi, Bluetooth and cell phone signals, and new ones are constantly being added. In view of this, it becomes even more important to find a "natural" area where you can walk

I know that for people who live in big cities, it isn't always easy to find a natural area close to home, but it should be possible to find a park that would at least be better than the air in the house or in your work place. On your days off, you can develop the new habit of finding yourself a healthier and more energizing space for walking.

A walk along the river, or a waterfall, or by the sea, enhances our immune system, as the movement of the water has the effect of cleansing our subtle bodies (mental and emotional) of their toxins.

Moving your arms while walking gives all your internal organs a massage and strengthens them as well. In other words, walking is without a doubt the best exercise for the body. It's a sport that is easy to do and, besides, it doesn't cost a penny. Walking is all the more important if you spend your day indoors and, especially, if you have a sedentary job.

*Wear brightly coloured clothing*

Are you someone who wears mainly black? If you are, it's your wound of rejection influencing you to do this, because you think it will help you suffer less: black prevents you from being in contact with your environment. But what you are forgetting is that others can't experience you either. People with the wound of injustice also generally prefer black, but for a different reason. They think it will make them appear thinner, which is very important to them. The fashion world has caught on to this preference and uses it to influence people more easily. The predominance of black in the fashion world serves to perpetuate and justify the existence of these two wounds.

**Everything that lives has a colour and every colour is associated with a different kind of energy.**

Did you know that all sounds and words emit a colour? The body is made up of the seven colours of the rainbow and we all need different colours to compensate for what is lacking in us, each day. We can pick up these colours then through what we wear, our contact with nature, the food we eat, etc. Have you ever thought how dull it would be if you were always served food that was black or if you lived in a house where the only colour around you was black? You should know that that is how your body feels when you choose to wear only black.

Many *Listen to Your Body* clients have gradually begun to wear colourful clothing and, in doing so, have been able to note amazing and marvellous changes in their life. By making the effort to wear more colour, and transforming your physical appearance in the process, you are initiating a psychological transformation. However, if you have already begun a transformation on the mental and emotional levels, it will be all the easier for you to add more colour to your wardrobe.

*Get more exposure to the sun*

The sun is a symbol of GOD. It represents life, energy, power, warmth, etc. Without sun, no form of life could exist on Earth. Could there be a connection between the fact that the pace at which people are living is constantly speeding up, with us spending our days at work and our evenings in front of the television or the computer (less sun exposure), and the fact that cancer rates are increasing? Some researchers answer in the affirmative.

I am writing this book in Mexico, by the ocean, and I cannot help but observe that for most people there is no balance about the amount of exposure they get to the sun. Indeed, most of them spend a good part of the year deprived of sunlight and then when they have the opportunity to spend time in a sunny place during their vacation time, they overdo it. They are exposed to the sun several hours a day, even at noon, when the sun's rays are, as everyone knows, at their strongest.

Being unaccustomed to such intense exposure, the body can only feel assaulted. This disrespectful attitude to the body is at the root of skin cancers which are an indication that the person has gone beyond their limits. It is likely that this person exercises a lot of control all year long and then, during vacation time, loses control and no longer recognizes their limits in various areas.

The ever-increasing incidence of these cancers is making people more fearful and this fear is in itself another factor contributing to the astounding increase seen over the last twenty years. This fear is doing us a lot of harm and, furthermore, it is not warranted. In fact less than 1% of people with skin cancer die from it, while a large percentage die from cancers associated with a lack of sun. Sunlight is essential for us because its ultraviolet B rays provide us with Vitamin D which aids in the absorption of calcium.

On a metaphysical level, the sun represents your inner GOD, as well as your light and your divine powers. Consequently, being exposed to the sun's rays in a balanced way shows you are in touch with your great power to create your life in a way that likewise is balanced. Otherwise, you are swinging the pendulum from the belief that you cannot create what you want, to a decision to want too much or to force things too quickly to be able to reach your goals, and your faith is definitely lacking in balance.

Why not combine your walks with getting some sun as often as you can, always keeping moderation in mind of course. I found out that 98% of the sunlight we absorb penetrates us through our eyes and that this light has a great energizing and healing power. We absorb the other 2% through our skin to produce Vitamin D, which, it would seem, strengthens our immune system and is known to help prevent cancer as well as autoimmune diseases.

I would therefore recommend that you wear sunglasses only when the glare of the sun is so strong that it prevents you from seeing clearly, when you are driving for example. Moreover, dark sunglasses could skew the message the body receives. Thinking it is in the shade, it may plausibly forget to multiply the cells on the surface layer of the skin to make it more impermeable to the sun's rays. And the body, believing it is in the shade, cannot stimulate the production of melanin which has the property of absorbing the high-energy ultraviolet B (UVB) rays and protecting the skin.

*Allow yourself small pleasures*

The greater your wound of rejection, the more difficult it is for you to offer yourself physical pleasure. When you buy something for yourself, it should not be only because you need it.

**Give yourself permission to buy something you do not really need, just for the pleasure of using it.**

Furthermore, why not start your day by saying, *What would it please me to do today?* Whatever the action, however small it may be, why not grant yourself the pleasure of it? You deserve several pleasures, large and small, every day. For example, you don't have to wait until you are tired or have a backache to treat yourself to a massage. In fact, this type of care is imperative for those suffering from rejection, as it helps develop your ability to be more sensitive to your body.

*Drink a lot of water*

This final recommendation is actually the most important. But unfortunately it is not sufficiently promoted in the Western world. On the contrary, this is not at all the case in the Eastern world, where medicine states that there are two principal causes of all health problems, whether physical or psychological. The first cause is microbes, bacteria and viruses while the second is the high rate of acidity caused by a lack of water.

I cannot get used to seeing, when I look around me, how little water people drink. I rarely meet anyone who drinks their two litres of water a day, which is nevertheless INDISPENSABLE for the proper functioning of the body. One should moreover not wait until one feels thirsty before drinking, because then the water is absorbed much too quickly and too much of it at once. The water passes right through you, just like with a dry plant that is heavily watered all at once and the water ends up flowing out onto the floor. The plant doesn't have time to absorb the water, just like our body which, very soon, needs to make its way to the toilet.

If you reply that you don't drink water because you are never thirsty, it indicates that your body has decided to stop letting you know its needs, because you haven't been listening to them for far too long. To regain the ability to sense thirst in your body, you need first of all to create a discipline. It will provide you with another great means of connecting more with your body, which will in turn help you to give it love.

It is also important to remember that the various other liquids you drink are not included in the two litres of water you need to drink. The water must be pure and natural in order to rid your body of the acid produced by almost everything we eat or drink now. These days all sorts of water with colour and additives is available on the market. All they do, especially the ones with sugar or sweetener added, is to produce more acid in your body. Do you love yourself enough to help your body? Choosing to harm your body is another indication of a lack of love for yourself.

## Loving yourself psychologically

The following suggestions offer you several ways you can help yourself on the psychological level.

*Be attentive to the thoughts you have*

Do your thoughts help guide you toward what you want to be or toward what you do not want to see happen in your life? When you can't sleep and your mind keeps replaying certain things that happened during the day, or stays focused on how rejected you felt by a family member or a friend, do these thoughts make you feel good? Perhaps your thoughts dwell on a certain person who often makes you feel rejected, but do you dare to express this or do you keep it to yourself?

I would remind you that because denial is such a frequent phenomenon among those suffering from rejection, you may very well be able to convince yourself that you are not experiencing rejection. And yet, there comes a time when you cannot stop thinking about the wrong another person has done to you, which is clearly a sign of great suffering. The more you ruminate over a long period, the greater your pain. Even if you tell yourself that you would like so much to be able to stop thinking about what hurts you, can you? If not, it is your wound of rejection that is making you so obsessive.

You would moreover like to have the courage to say what you think to those who have hurt you but do not succeed. Have you noticed that when you entertain such thoughts, the situation worsens, because your imagination ends up distorting reality? And your imagination is influenced by the parts in you that suffer, as well as by your ego which has been able to get the upper hand due to the fear you experience. If you could instead envision making peace with these persons, it would trigger an act of love toward yourself.

When you read about the research and discoveries of the Japanese doctor, Masaro Emoto, you can understand the power of thought. In fact, he has proven beyond any doubt, by means of remarkable photos, how much a person can affect the quality of water merely through their thoughts or words. Knowing that our body is composed of 65% water, which is the symbol of our emotional body, lets us immediately grasp how much our emotions, especially hatred and bitterness, influence the health of our body.

That's why it is so important to remain in charge of your thoughts and feelings rather than letting them be influenced by all the negative things you have learned or by the remarks and beliefs of others. I'm thinking of a woman who had to see her doctor for some test results following the discovery of a lump in one of her breasts. As she was fearful about the outcome, she asked her daughter – who was pregnant with her first child – to accompany her. The doctor asked the usual questions about the family history, whether her mother or any of the other women in the family had ever had cancer, etc. When she replied that there had never been cancer in the family, that no one, including her sisters, had ever had cancer, the doctor turned to the woman's daughter and said, *Well, madame, now that you know your mother has cancer, be prepared. You are now a good candidate for having it too. Be very careful in the future and be sure to have regular checkups.*

Mother and daughter left the doctor's office in a state of shock, even though they were aware that this doctor was someone who believed firmly in the statistics and that it was not his intention to frighten them. Knowing full well the power of thought, the mother had to be very clear with her daughter that she should not trust blindly in what she had just heard.

Remember that you can never control what others believe or say, but you can on the other hand decide to be totally in charge of your own thoughts and consequently of your words, which are always a reflection of what you think.

*Get restorative sleep*

Are you aware that your subconscious repeats all night the last thought you had before falling asleep? That's why people are always advised against reading books or watching movies with violence in them, or even worse, listening to all the bad news of the day on the radio or television before going to bed. So many people even have a TV in their bedroom and sometimes fall asleep with a violent scene being the last image they see.

Poor mental body! It does not have a chance to regenerate during the night, which is the main purpose of sleep. Why? Because during sleep, your subtle bodies – your emotional and mental bodies – need to leave your physical body, thus giving your three bodies a chance to rest and regenerate. The more the mental body is agitated and anxious during the night, the more the subtle bodies have trouble detaching themselves. This explains why certain people know they have slept several hours but wake up just as tired if not more so than the night before.

Others, who fall asleep in front of the TV while it is still on, have the impression they do not sleep. Their subtle bodies detach themselves, but remain very close to the physical body instead of going off to be regenerated in other spheres, and this explains the fact that these people hear in the distance what is happening on the television screen. The person's subconscious absorbs everything being said on TV, while they are sleeping.

So, before going to sleep, it is therefore an excellent idea to immerse yourself in some inspiring reading. It has the advantage of being able to raise your vibration levels of love and self-esteem, even if only for five minutes. If despite everything, you have difficulty falling asleep due to a lot of mental activity that you can't manage to halt – worries, obsessions, emotions, etc. – the best way is to get up and write down everything that goes through your head. Then end your list with what you want the outcome of this situation to be. When you get back into bed, visualize only the things that you want.

You can also repeat a sentence that expresses clearly what you want to see happen, for example, *I see Sophie's good intention in what she said to me today* or *I tell my boss about the problem I am having with him, which I have not dared to tell him before*. If you can visualize yourself actually manifesting and experiencing the happiness of achieving such a goal by repeating these sentences, that visualization process will give you the energy you need to get there.

Your subconscious will work for you by repeating to you all night whatever you said before going to sleep. Do not be surprised to wake up with a solution to your problems. I remind you however that it is very important to respect your limits. Even if you must repeat sentences like this for weeks before you have success, at least you are creating mental and emotional reinforcement day by day.

If you are suffering from a cancerous tumour at this time, add the visualization of this tumour bathed in a pool of light and the sparkling sensation the light produces. Allow your divine light to energize you, for it is in contact with the needs of your soul.

*Say thank you*

What an important word! Have you ever noticed how many times in a day you say thank you to others? And what about yourself? Do you thank yourself? I am certain that you say thank you more often to others than to yourself, while what should happen is just the opposite. Why? Because with the wounds of rejection and injustice, it is normal to be perfectionist and demanding and to feel you need to do something exceptional before praising yourself or thinking of saying thank you. Since you will lack a bit of practice, it is normal that you should find this more difficult at first.

I'm sure you know that the more you practise something new, the easier it gets to assimilate it and apply it. It is said a new habit must be practised for at least three months before the brain can successfully establish the new connections needed to make it easier. You may have to set up some kind of signal, on the hour for example, as a reminder. Or you could place a little note near your bed to help you think of saying thank you to yourself for at least three things that day before you go to sleep. That way you will learn to thank yourself more and more often and attract an increasing number of pleasant experiences into your life.

**We should not say thank you only because we have just received something, we receive more and more BECAUSE we say thank you.**

*See the quality in a fault*

This involves starting to be more conscious of what you consider "your qualities and your faults." I am thinking for example of the people who have the "fault" of answering too quickly and saying hurtful things. They consider it a fault but actually it's the other side of their quality of being quick-witted. This quality is applied in the wrong context because they have been holding back too much, being influenced by their fear of rejection.

Take the time then to make a list of what you consider to be "your faults." Then note down beside each of them the quality you must have if you demonstrate this fault. You will become conscious that it was quite simply not being used in the right context and in the right manner. By giving yourself the right to not always know how to use this quality, you will gradually learn to use it more appropriately and in the way you wish.

*See only beauty*

Beauty is the emotional body's greatest need. Make sure you surround yourself only with items that you find beautiful and remember that "beauty" is not synonymous with "expensive." You don't need to spend a fortune to be surrounded by beauty. As soon as one of your possessions seems faded or dull, give it away, sell it or throw it out, to make room for something new. The following task will definitely help you in the next few days: take a tour of your home and check what you find beautiful about each object. It is said that an intelligent person acquires only things that offer them at least one use. You should know that beauty is very useful indeed.

So many people keep masses of old things just because they are still usable, even if they do not bring any use or beauty into their lives. I am thinking of an elderly couple where one of them wanted to change the living room furniture, which was thirty years old, but the other refused because it was still in good condition and served perfectly well. Ten years later, they still have the same living room furniture. Why deprive oneself of this small joy which could nourish the emotional body, if one can easily afford it financially?

To know what you find beautiful, you need to be sensitive to beauty. Beauty is thus an excellent tool for developing your sensitivity, just like music is. Not only does everything that lives have colour, as mentioned above, but all sounds have a colour too. If you listen to rhythmic music and cannot feel it and let your body move, it is because you are too cut off from your environment. Let me remind you that one of the best ways to heal the wound of rejection is to be able to feel that you are part of the great all. If you feel alone and separate from your environment, it is due to your own decision. No one has the power to cut you off from your surroundings – except you.

*Take life less seriously*

This involves learning to let go and laugh more, and taking yourself less seriously.

**Letting go means being fine with the outcome of a situation, even when it does not coincide with what you had hoped for. It is impossible to control everything.**

In fact, the term "control" is the exact opposite of letting go. If you have confidence in your inner GOD, who always knows what you need, then even if a person or a situation is in sharp contrast with your expectations, you will feel assured that there is a good reason for this and that you will become aware of it in due course. You will become aware of it when you are able to take responsibility and see that this situation or this person was able to teach you something. I like the saying **"let go and let God take over".**

As stated in Chapter Two regarding DNA, it has been proven that laughter brings countless benefits, the main one being the ability to strengthen the immune system. *Laughter therapy* has been around for several years now and there have been innumerable cures attributed to it. If you have trouble finding life funny, why not rent comedy movies to help you out?

Before being able to laugh at situations, or to laugh at yourself instead of rejecting yourself, I suggest smiling more. Even if you have nothing to smile about at the moment, force yourself to smile with your lips and gradually you will be able to smile with your eyes too. Have you ever noticed the effect a beautiful smile coming from another person has on you? Know that your own smile has the same effect on you and on others. Remember that it is just for yourself that you are acting this way and that you amply deserve to adopt new habits that will make you feel better.

*Live your present moment*

You know you are living your present moment when you take the time to really appreciate what is happening in the present moment. If you impose on yourself for example a certain way of walking or eating everyday in the hope of healing through such action, you are not in your present moment, but rather, in the future. The aim is not so much to be healed as it is to live many small joys every minute.

**Happiness can only be present in the "here and now."**

When you run away from a situation or when you are in denial, so that you don't have to take the time to feel, you are certainly not in your present moment, any more than you are when you have expectations. Most sick people, moreover, live in expectation: they wait for test results and for surgery and for the outcome of the surgery; they expect attention from their family and friends as well as understanding from others; they hope to regain their energy; they await the news that they are finally better... and news of a probable relapse.

When you find you are afraid, the fastest and most effective way to come back into your present moment, is to take several deep breaths, feel the fear for yourself in this situation (or the fear for yourself with regard to someone else) and quite simply authorize yourself to be afraid at this time. Afterwards, ask yourself what it is you want for this situation and turn your attention and your energy toward this positive goal, rather than to what you do not want to see happen.

**Every visualization based on self-love and on your needs – and not on a fear – is automatically manifested according to the level of what you feel at that precise moment.**

You will realize afterwards just how effective this kind of acceptance is in reconnecting you with your great power to create the life you want. Let me remind you that this notion of acceptance, which is a spiritual notion, is not always easy to put into practice because of the interference of the ego. But if you develop the good habit of accepting your fears as they show up, you will succeed more and more easily. You will also more quickly develop the ability to appreciate everything around you. It is impossible for anyone to experience only unpleasant moments in their life. What do you choose to give your attention to?

*Have goals*

It is important to set goals for yourself to help guide you toward what you want. What are your short-term goals, your more long-term goals? Do you know what you want, what would please you? And above all, do not forget this: what will the manifestation of your desire help you to BE?

Here is what you must retain: your desires and your goals must always be at the service of what you want to be. You must not wait until you are sure all the circumstances are perfect before you give yourself permission to set a goal, for you would surely miss several good opportunities. This is an attitude often seen in perfectionists. They think that not reaching a goal represents failure, which makes them reject themselves even more and persuades them that there is no point in continuing to have goals.

But your heart says the opposite. It tells you, among other things, to have several goals in your life and to move toward them by letting go. And this is easily done when you have confidence in your inner power, which always sends you what you need when you need it. Having goals, looking forward to things, wanting to get up in the morning at the thought of aiming for something that goes WOW inside you, these are excellent foods for your emotional body and they fill you with energy. A person without a goal is dying a slow death, as they fail to nourish their emotional body.

There is nothing to prevent you from taking steps toward what you want, but always remember that if it doesn't happen, it's only because there is something better for you that awaits. You must especially remember that YOU ARE NOT A FAILURE, YOU ARE NOT WHAT YOU DO. You are a spiritual being who is on Earth to have experiences.

**You could say that in life, there are no failures or mistakes, there are only experiences to help us learn about ourselves.**

Actually, our ego does not know that we must experience everything in order to finally be able to accept ourselves in all our aspects, positive as well as negative.

*Dare to express yourself more*

The worse the illness you are facing – even possibly a life-threatening illness –, the more urgent it is for you to express yourself. Dare to talk about yourself, about what you feel in your deepest self, rather than thinking that what you have to say could not possibly be of interest to anyone. Even if it feels awkward at first, remember that everything gets easier with practice.

Your motivation for expressing yourself must however be to help you become liberated from what you are experiencing and not to be understood by others. Others have the right in any event to not understand you or even be interested in what you have to say. You should first see if the other person is willing to take some time to listen to you. That's all. Remember however that they have no obligation to agree to listen to you.

**If someone says no, they are not rejecting you, they are just expressing their own need.**

If they aren't willing, you are receiving the message to find another person of whom you can make the same request. It is your inner GOD who knows there is someone else who will meet your need better. You need then to find that person but in order to succeed, you need to speak up and make your intent known.

Regarding the manner in which you express yourself, pay attention to the words you use, such as *"my cancer," "I'll never be able to..," "I'm afraid of a relapse,"* and so forth.

Why not replace them with "cancer," "I'm gradually learning to...," "I'm giving my body the time it needs to return to its natural state"? Can you feel the difference between these two ways of expressing yourself through the kinds of sensations they produce in you?

Remember that the subconscious works only with images associated with the words you use. When for example you say, *"I'm fed up with being sick,"* or *"I don't want to be sick anymore,"* your subconscious sees or perceives the images of a sick person. To make it easier for your subconscious, you need to affirm what you want in a positive way, being especially attentive to avoid sentences containing NOT.

*Change the label*

It is sad to see how many people suffering from one type of illness or another get labelled under some general term and put into a category, as if the illness were something irreversible. *My brother-in-law is a cancer patient, a heart patient* or *an asthmatic,* or *an alcoholic,* or *bipolar,* etc.

And what about you? Have you labelled yourself too? Every time you think or say, *I am sick,* you believe you are your illness. Remember that you ARE NOT your cancer.

**You ARE NOT your illness, you ARE a very powerful divine being.**

If you have had the power to create an illness, a cancer, etc., why not use that same power to free yourself from it? Instead of saying, *"I am sick,"* why not say, *"I suffer"* or *"I have a cancer problem or cancerous cells right now"*? Don't forget to add, RIGHT NOW, for everything on this planet is temporary. Only you have the power to make your illness permanent, based on your choice and your decision.

**In reality, cancer is not fatal, cancer is a message you receive from your inner GOD who only wants happiness and inner peace for you.**

Cancer is an opportunity given to you for your transformation, to help you love yourself more. How you perceive this word is entirely your responsibility.

Families also get labelled: *a family with heart disease, a family with a history of cancer, depression runs in their family,* etc. It is true that members of the same family tend to be born with similar life paths, similar beliefs and wounds. But you don't need to think that because there is a history of cancer in your family, you will inevitably experience it too. Such a belief serves only to generate fear and it is this fear, rather, that will be the cause of a potential cancer. You have the power to continue to believe in statistics, scientific hypotheses and popular beliefs... or to believe that you ARE NOT your physical body and that you are much more than that.

We know that science conceives illness as an organic or functional change in the body and that its approach is based on statistics and hypotheses.

**Statistics are not prognoses (judgment regarding the progress of an illness) or indicators of terminal illness. It is believing in them that makes the illness terminal.**

Too often, the goal of medicine is to make the disease disappear. This is why so many doctors treat only the symptoms.

## The power to heal

Why not decide right now that by changing your way of thinking, by reconciling with your parents, by accepting yourself completely as you are, you give yourself the power to change your future and not give in to general or family statistics. Let me repeat: you are the only one with this power.

Doctors will never guarantee a cure, for they know full well that the same treatment can have good results in one person and mediocre results, or even none, in the next person. When you hurt yourself, the doctor can of course put in stitches or prescribe an ointment or medication. However, you know very well that that's not all that healed your wound. It is your body with all its healing power that, in the end, did the real work of healing.

**Medicine has the power to treat, but it is the acceptance of what you ARE that truly heals.**

More and more doctors subscribe to this theory. They even go as far as prescribing placebo medications to their patients. This was even being done as early as the 18th century. According to a study done in 2008, 45% of American doctors working in a hospital prescribe placebo medications, but only 4% of them tell their patients. The percentage of people reported to experience improvement following the placebo medication is 39%, which is virtually the same percentage as for those who receive a morphine injection without their knowledge. Doctors also did a study to find out if there was a specific personality type more likely to respond to a placebo. The results were inconclusive.

An interesting fact: it has been proven that doctors or therapists who take the time to really listen to their patients, and who believe that the power to be completely healed is in their hands, present much better results with placebo medications. This shows that the patient who senses how much their doctor believes in the patient's power to heal has a much easier time believing in the benefits of the medication. It is thus a combination of the doctor's empathetic listening, on the one hand, and both parties believing in the healing, on the other, that can produce such remarkable results.

The natural world of plants and animals, including the human body, constitutes the most sophisticated and impressive pharmacy we know of. First of all, it is free. Our body's ability to automatically secrete endorphins as soon as we feel happy serves as a good example. It represents something less expensive and less harmful than morphine. The good news is that we are the only species on Earth that has the power to decide to be happy. And what about you? Do you choose to be happy or unhappy?

It has also been proven that regular physical activity (brisk walking, cycling, swimming, etc.) for at least thirty minutes a day at a sustained pace, increases the natural production of endorphins, the same hormones that are released naturally after orgasm. But we need also to be aware that endorphins deteriorate rapidly and their beneficial effect is short-lived. It is therefore important to give yourself pleasure as often as possible and to always try to find the bright side of a situation.

It is interesting to note that, being affected by their wound of rejection in the area of sexuality, many people have difficulty reaching orgasm, and it is not because of a lack of sensitivity. On the contrary, they are very sensitive but think themselves not worthy enough for permission to enjoy this great physical pleasure. If this sounds like you, don't despair over it, for the ability to reach orgasm can be discovered at any age. You have only to decide on it and grant yourself the right. Why wouldn't you be entitled to experience this incredible sensation of wellbeing that nature offers you through the release of endorphins?

It has also been observed that a significant number of animals heal faster than humans do, from the same disorder, and some are even able to re-grow a severed limb. How can this be explained? Animals are not afraid and have complete trust in what their body can do, even if it is unconsciously. Animals are natural and have no ego. When we let nature's intelligence follow its course, miracles can happen.

I have had the privilege of hearing thousands of testimonies from people recounting how quickly they were able to heal following an accident because they had understood the spiritual message of the incident. For example, someone breaks a leg in two places and gets a plaster cast. When they visit the doctor three weeks later, they find out that everything has healed and the cast is no longer necessary. Doctors are often very surprised when they observe these kinds of phenomena. Most are quite happy to note them, even if they cannot understand how a person can heal in three weeks instead of in the three months anticipated. The human body is the most extraordinary creation that exists on our planet. The more we become conscious of this, the more we will be in love with this highly complex and oh-so-marvellous instrument. It makes us want nothing more than to keep it happy as much as possible.

If however you think it is impossible for you to heal, or if you attract illnesses in order to have attention, you are going against the great laws of self-love, and your chances of healing drop significantly.

Here is another example about a broken leg, but with a different outcome. A woman sustained two fractures in her leg from a car accident. She needed surgery because they were not clean breaks. Her doctor told her however that she should be able to walk again and go back to work in six months at the outside. After half a year, her leg did not seem to want to heal as it was supposed to. After another hospital stay and several examinations, she was told that everything was fine, that the operation had been a success and that there was no reason why her leg was not healing as it ought to.

The message this woman was receiving through this accident, but which she did not want to see, was that she was feeling guilty about not wanting to go back to work. She did not dare tell her husband this, or give herself permission for it, as both of them would have had to rein in significantly the lifestyle they were used to. The spiritual message was that she should allow herself to be afraid to let go of her job and at the same time, stop feeling guilty about not wanting to work anymore. If she had accepted her fear at that time, she could have kept on working and felt much better about it, or alternatively, actually stopped working, but with greater confidence. Who knows? She could have attracted a situation allowing her to find a different job that was physically less demanding or another unexpected source of income.

When she learned that her insurance would pay 80% of her salary for five years, she continued to limp around and use a crutch for all of that time, without doctors being able to do anything to help her. In the weeks following termination of the payout period, her leg wasted no time in healing and she started back to work.

Do you see just how much a person's intention or motivation can completely change their life? How will you make your choices for your future? Will you be motivated by fear and reap results that are far from beneficial, or by love for yourself, which will guide you toward increased wellbeing?

I could cite numerous examples similar to that one. In short, this woman preferred to suffer for five years to be able to feel entitled to what she wanted, while she could have used her power to create what she wanted without suffering. When I witness or hear these stories, I always marvel at the power of a human being to either heal themselves or bring sickness upon themselves.

**It is the same energy you use to guide yourself toward what you want or toward what you don't want. Which is the more intelligent choice to make?**

## Accepting death = accepting life

I have just been speaking to you in the section above about our immense power to heal, but that decision to live must be accompanied by an acceptance of death. I have already spoken about the fear of death in Chapter Seven but I want to return to the topic now because it is a very important part of life to accept. Those who do not accept death are acting as if they are immortal, and are not showing respect for life. I have known many of them who, even when they are suffering from a serious illness, do not what to hear any talk of death. Some even refuse to make a will, saying they are still too young for that. That kind of attitude comes from selfishness and a lack of responsibility. They seem to think that it is normal for their loved ones to have to assume all the unpleasant consequences of a deceased person not leaving a last will and testament – consequences resulting from their decision and not the decision of their family and friends.

**Death is not a punishment, nor is it a failure, it is only a passage to another dimension.**

Death is necessary in order to allow us to take stock with regard to what has just taken place in the last life, and prepare us for the next. We may compare it to a night of sleep allowing us to refuel for the next day. It is a natural stage in life. There are even several doctors who are afraid of death, who still believe that they have failed whenever they see one of their patients die. I have always thought that the first thing that should be taught at medical school is how to help patients accept death, even as they opt to live.

If you are someone who is afraid to talk about the fact that you or someone close to you might die, it means that you are equally afraid to live. You are not living for yourself, you are living to carry out your duty or to make others happy. You must also often have the impression of having to struggle in life. Thus you do not manage to follow your life path and will have to return to Earth to start all over again.

You could compare this attitude to that of students who do not do any of their school assignments and have therefore to repeat the same grade or course. In reality, they are the only losers in this decision and are not punishing anyone other than themselves – by orienting themselves to what they do not want, rather than toward what they do want in life.

If you have trouble accepting the idea of dying one day, or that one of your loved ones may die, is it possible that you believe that accepting the idea of death is equivalent to choosing to abdicate life? Do you think it means you are choosing not to want to live any longer? If so, tell yourself firmly that it is your ego making you believe such things. Your ego is convinced that accepting means submitting, being resigned to something. It is normal for your ego to believe that, because it is incapable of understanding any spiritual notion.

Accepting death as a phase of life, just as sleep is part of the activity of the day, will help you to let go of any bitterness, hatred or obsessions you may have. When you do experience emotions due to feelings of rejection, it will be easier for you to have the following reaction: If I should happen to die tomorrow, in what state would I like to leave? In one of continued resentment toward others or one of peace and reconciliation?

This acceptance will help you moreover to know that you are on earth to learn to live in unconditional love and discover the extraordinary being that you are, that is, a divine being. You will then know just how beneficial reconciliation and forgiveness are, for they answer the needs of your soul.

The more you reconnect with the true love that lives in you, the more your inner light will shine in you and around you. You may compare life to a huge warehouse without light. You walk around inside this warehouse with your flashlight. From time to time, you can see other people walking around with their own flashlight. You can only see what your flashlight illuminates and you can only identify things based on the limited knowledge you have.

With so little light, if you are looking for something specific – which might represent happiness or health, for example – it could take a very long time before you find it. So, does that mean that if you don't find a certain object in that warehouse, it doesn't exist? Well, life is like that. As your light begins to expand through the love you develop, you come to realize that life is quite different from the limited picture you had imagined before. Imagine all the lights in the warehouse turned on! That's what it will be like when you are filled with love for yourself.

## Collective healing

We learned from *Carl Gustav Jung,* the famous psychiatrist, physician and psychologist whom I mentioned earlier, that we are all part of a collective unconsciousness. Indeed he was the first to do extensive research in this area and make discoveries regarding "archetypes," "the collective unconscious," and "synchronicity." In short, his idea was that all thoughts and all feelings experienced by each one of us are also sensed by all living things on this planet. This can explain why a dog's attitude is the reflection of the master's attitude, why a flower offered and received with love lasts much longer, etc.

When I learned this, my first reaction was to say to myself that if the natural world of plants and animals can perceive everything unconsciously, surely the human race must all the more be able to perceive all things not only unconsciously, but consciously as well. Our conscious awareness is proving to be the most manifest consciousness on Earth.

Since love and hate are the strongest sentiments, imagine the effect we might be having, not just on our immediate surroundings, but also throughout the earth, if we decide to continue to hate rather than to love, love representing the natural state of all living things.

Take the example of a glass you want to fill with water. Every thought contrary to love is like a drop of dirty water put into the glass, and every loving thought a drop of pure water. How do you perceive your glass? Full of pure or impure water? Truly, it is never too late to change the way you act. Every time you carry out an act of love toward yourself or toward another, by welcoming without attaching judgment, you are adding pure water. Then you can know with certainty that the water in the glass will be purified little by little.

Each person's glass of water fills an immense glass which represents the state of all living things on Earth. Every act, whether it is one of love, acceptance, hate, bitterness or fear, contributes to the general state of the planet. What is the most intelligent choice? To foster the life of this home where we live or to destroy it?

Since people suffering from the wound of rejection believe they are alone and isolated from the rest of the world, it takes extra effort for them to be able to accept that they have a great influence on the rest of the planet. How do you see yourself? Do you make yourself believe that because you often have people around you, you do not feel isolated? I am talking about FEELING alone, not about what's happening in your environment.

If this is you, why not write yourself a little note reminding you that each of your thoughts and emotions are felt by those close to you and by the rest of the planet, and put it in a visible place in your home? Why not also put one at your place of work? That way, you will begin to return to your natural state, which is to know and feel that you are part of the great whole. It would be ridiculous if each drop of water or each wave in the sea thought it was separate. It will be easier for you, then, to start opening up and talking about your feelings.

If a doctor or therapist treats only the sick part, they continue to encourage this sense of isolation and dissociation from the rest of the world, which is what our ego does too. Quantum physics clearly tells us that everything is made of atoms that communicate with each other. It is therefore your responsibility to choose someone who will help you *holistically*. This kind of approach will afford you the best chance of being able to return to your natural state of being healthy again.

## Healing the wound of rejection

By putting into practice what has been suggested in this book with regard to loving yourself, you are contributing to healing your wound of rejection. When you do this, your physical body will feel the effects, since it is the reflection of what is going on in you. If you read this book and do not suffer from cancer or any other illness, learning to love yourself more is the most effective way to prevent any health problem. I would remind you however that this is not achieved in a few days. Relearning to love yourself is done gradually and each time your body lets you know about a health problem, it will be a gift for you, for your body is only trying to draw your attention to a situation where you have forgotten to love and accept yourself.

Instead of letting your wound of rejection control your life, instead of letting your fears, obsessions and sense of inferiority eat away at you, instead of letting your wound of rejection isolate you from others and keep you from taking your rightful place, you will return to your natural self, and here is what it will look like! You are

- gifted with resilience at work and are able to handle a lot;
- resourceful and have a talent for creativity, inventiveness and imagination;
- capable of working alone or together with others, equally comfortable in either situation;

- able to respond appropriately and do what is required in an emergency;
- able to withdraw, without feeling diminished;
- more realistic in how you see the world;
- more connected to what is going on around you;
- able to give your opinion while understanding that others have the right to disagree;
- aware that if others say no, they are only expressing their limits;
- able to distinguish between what you do and what you ARE.

To summarize, isn't it marvellous to know that you have everything you need to heal yourself both physically and psychologically? It is up to you to decide, and to desire it with your whole being. This great power that lives within you is just waiting to be discovered.

**What will you decide today? To guide your steps toward what you want to be, and live? Or walk in the opposite direction?**

If you would like to be notified when Lise Bourbeau's next book is released, send us your contact information...

... by e-mail: info@leseditionsetc.com

... by fax: 450-431-0991

... by mail:

Les Éditions ETC
1102 Boul. La Salette
St-Jérôme (Québec)
J5L 2J7 CANADA

# The BE yourself workshop

The dynamic and practical teachings of the BE YOURSELF workshop can help all those who really want to IMPROVE their quality of life. This one of a kind opportunity provides you with a solid foundation to pursue what you want out of life.

The workshop is divided into two different days* in Canada, and you can choose to participate in one or both sessions.

Day 1 **BE YOUR TRUE SELF**
by letting go of what you believe you should be

Come find out what your current needs are and how to satisfy them in order to feel good and be happy. Step by step, you will discover a number of different tools, including the important step of discovering how much you really love yourself.

**You will learn, among other things, how to...**

- identify the fears and beliefs which serve as stumbling blocks to your happiness;
- discover what is preventing you from being who you want to be;
- deal with dissatisfaction and reach serenity;
- use the tools that are simple and necessary to be in harmony with yourself.

**Dare to take the first step and come learn how to be yourself!**

# Find us on f

**Join the LISE BOURBEAU READERS CLUB**
**and chat with members from**
**around the world.**

We created a Facebook Group to bring together people from around the world who have a common interest in Lise Bourbeau's books and workshops.

Our primary intention is to offer YOU the opportunity to share your ideas, questions, and advice to other members of this group based on the Listen To Your Body philosophy, created by Lise Bourbeau.

# Books from the same author

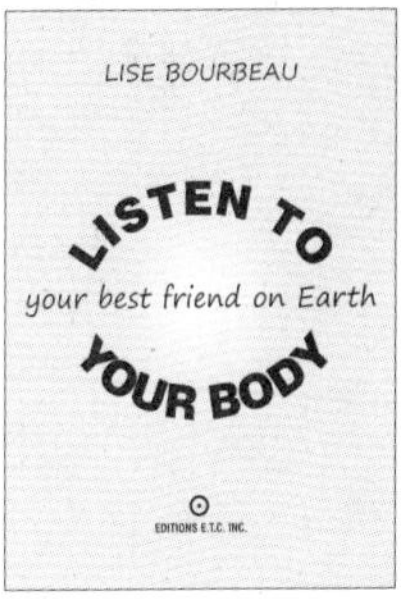


***Listen to your best friend on Earth, your body***

LISE BOURBEAU takes you by the hand and, step by step, leads you beyond "packing your own parachute", to taking that step back into the clear, refreshing stream of life that flows from the Universal Source. She gives you the tools, not only to fix what is wrong in your life, but to build a solid foundation for your inner house - a foundation that extends as far as the global village. In this book, she helps you build an intimate, rewarding and powerful relationship with the most important person in your life - yourself.

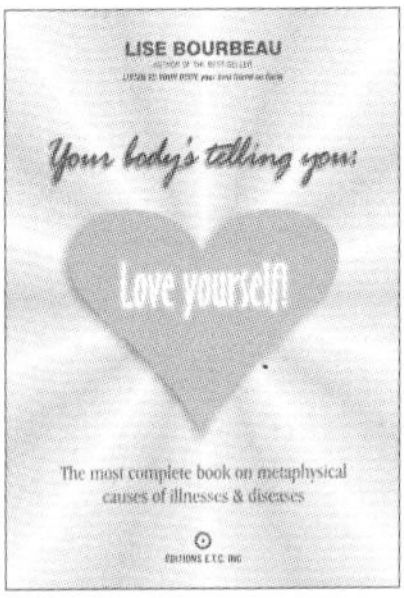


***Your body's telling you: Love yourself!***

Lise Bourbeau has compiled 20 years of research in the field of metaphysics and it's physical manifestations in the body and brought it all to the forefront in this user-friendly reference guide, Your body's telling you: Love yourself! Since 1982, she has worked successfully with over 15,000 people, helping them to unearth the underlying causes of specific illnesses and diseases. A comprehensive guide to the metaphysical causes of over 500 illnesses and diseases, is a succinct and visionary work that is truly and literally a labor of love.

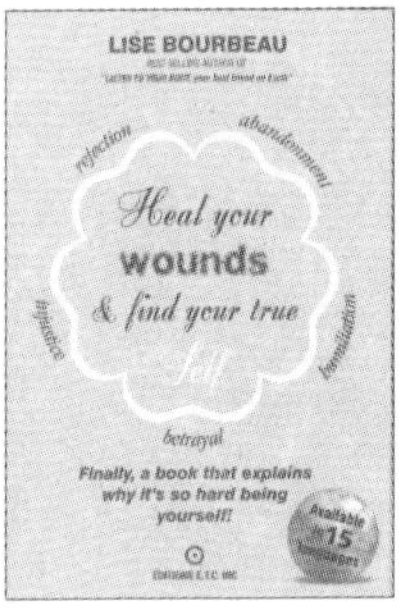


***Heal your wounds and find your true self***

Do you sometimes feel that you are going around in circles in your personal growth? Do you occasionally see a problem re-emerge, thinking you had solved it? Perhaps it's because you're not looking in the right place.

This new book by Lise Bourbeau, as concrete as her others, demonstrates that all problems, whether physical, emotional or mental, stem from five important wounds: *rejection, abandonment, humiliation, betrayal* and *injustice*. This book contains detailed descriptions of these wounds and of the masks we've developed to hide them.

This book will allow you to set off on the path that leads to complete healing, the path that leads to your ultimate goal: your true self.

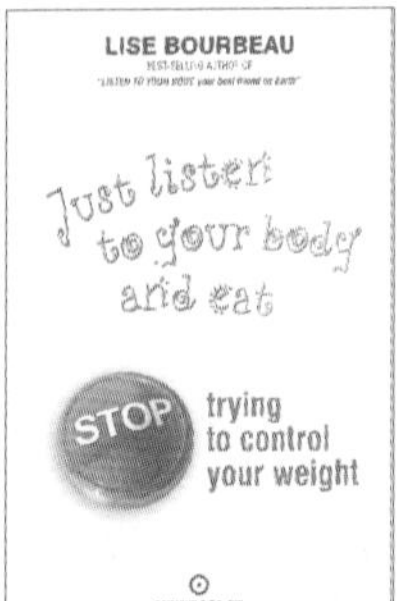


***Just listen to your body and eat - STOP trying to control your weight***

Lise Bourbeau's new book has many goals:

... help you discover that there are six reasons besides hunger that make you want to eat; ... show you how much you control your food intake and how that can be bad for you; ... teach you to quickly recognize the emotional wounds that prevent you from eating well; and help you love and accept your body, and especially who you are at every moment.

This eagerly awaited book offers an entirely new way of looking at your relationship with your food. It reveals the connection between the physical, emotional, mental and spiritual dimensions of the person and can help you, in this way, to discover your own specific needs at any given time.

# 3 ways to order

| TITLE | QTY. | TOTAL |
| --- | --- | --- |
| | | |
| | | |
| | | |
| | | |
| | | |
| | | |
| | | |
| | | |
| | | |
| | | |
| | | |
| | | |
| | | |
| | SUB-TOTAL | |
| | SHIPPING | |
| | **TOTAL** | |

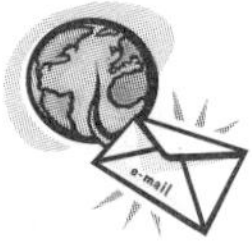


info@listentoyourbody.net

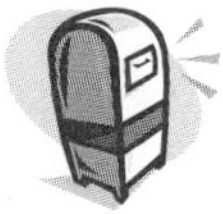

ECOUTE TON CORPS
1102 La Salette Blv
St-Jerome (Quebec)
J5L 2J7 CANADA

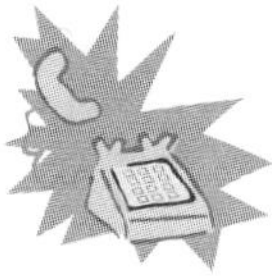

**1-800-361-3834**
**or 450-431-5336**

SHIPPING & HANDLING FEES
CANADA and US : 12$CAN
INTERNATIONAL: contact us

VISA Number: ____ Exp.: __ / __ (month / year)

MasterCard Cardholder's name: ____

Signature: ____

CANADIAN MONEY ORDER made out to ECOUTE TON CORPS

e: ____

ess: ____

Town - State/Province: ____ Zip code: ____

hone #: ( ) ____ Country ____